HEALTH-CARE SYSTEMS
CUMULATIVE INDEX

9

Health-Care Systems
Cumulative Index

MACMILLAN LIBRARY REFERENCE USA
Simon & Schuster Macmillan
NEW YORK

Simon & Schuster and Prentice Hall International
LONDON · MEXICO CITY · NEW DELHI · SINGAPORE · SYDNEY · TORONTO

MACMILLAN

HEALTH

ENCYCLOPEDIA

9

EDITORIAL CREDITS

Developed and produced by
Visual Education Corporation, Princeton, NJ

Project Editor: Darryl Kestler

Editors: Richard Bohlander, Susan Garver,
Michael Gee, Emilie McCardell,
Cynthia Mooney, Suzanne Murdico,
Frances Wiser

Editorial Assistant: Carol Ciaston

Photo Editors: Maryellen Costa, Michael Gee

Photo Research: Cynthia Cappa, Sara Matthews

Production Supervisor: Anita Crandall

Proofreading Management: Amy Davis

Art Editors: Maureen Pancza, Mary Lyn Sodano

Advisor, Anatomical Illustrations:
David Seiden, Ph.D.
Robert Wood Johnson Medical School
Piscataway, New Jersey

Layout: Maxson Crandall, Lisa Evans

Word Processing: Cynthia Feldner

Design: Hespenheide Design

The information contained in the *Macmillan Health Encyclopedia* is not intended to take the place of the care and advice of a physician or health-care professional. Readers should obtain professional advice in making health-care decisions.

PHOTO CREDITS

Jacket: Howard Sochurek/The Stock Market

Brooklyn Image Group: Lorraine Corsale, 18; Curtis Willocks, 39

PhotoEdit: 27; Vic Bider, 12; Robert Brenner, 7; Paul Conklin, 24 (right); Tony Freeman, 10, 15, 30; Dennis MacDonald, 24 (left); Elena Rooraid, 28; Dave Schaefer, 22; James Shaffer, 20; Susan Van Etten, 23; David Young-Wolff, 36

The Picture Cube: L. S. Stepanowicz, 37

SIU: Visuals Unlimited, 5

Terry Wild Studio: 6, 40

Visuals Unlimited: John D. Cunningham, 19

SIMON & SCHUSTER MACMILLAN
Macmillan Library Reference
1633 Broadway
New York, NY 10019-6785

Printed in the United States of America

printing number
10 9 8 7 6 5 4 3

Library of Congress Cataloging-in-Publication Data
Macmillan health encyclopedia.
    v. <1–   >
    Includes index.
    Contents: v. 1. Body systems—v. 2. Communicable diseases—v. 3. Noncommunicable diseases and disorders—v. 4 Nutrition and fitness—v. 5. Emotional and mental health—v. 6. Sexuality and reproduction—v. 7. Drugs, alcohol, and tobacco—v. 8. Safety and environmental health—v. 9. Health-care systems/cumulative index
    ISBN 0-02-897439-5 (set).—ISBN 0-02-897431-X (v. 1).—ISBN 0-02-897432-8 (v. 2).
    1. Health—Encyclopedias.   I. Macmillan Publishing Company.
RA776.M174   1993
610´ .3—dc20
                                           92-28939
                                               CIP

Volumes of the *Macmillan Health Encyclopedia*

1 *Body Systems* (ISBN 0-02-897431-X)
2 *Communicable Diseases* (ISBN 0-02-897432-8)
3 *Noncommunicable Diseases and Disorders* (ISBN 0-02-897433-6)
4 *Nutrition and Fitness* (ISBN 0-02-897434-4)
5 *Emotional and Mental Health* (ISBN 0-02-897435-2)
6 *Sexuality and Reproduction* (ISBN 0-02-897436-0)
7 *Drugs, Alcohol, and Tobacco* (ISBN 0-02-897437-9)
8 *Safety and Environmental Health* (ISBN 0-02-897438-7)
9 *Health-Care Systems/Cumulative Index* (ISBN 0-02-897453-0)

PREFACE

The *Macmillan Health Encyclopedia* is a nine-volume set that explains how the body works; describes the causes and treatment of hundreds of diseases and disorders; provides information on diet and exercise for a healthy lifestyle; discusses key issues in emotional, mental, and sexual health; covers problems relating to the use and abuse of legal and illegal drugs; outlines first-aid procedures; and provides up-to-date information on current health issues.

Written with the support of a distinguished panel of editorial advisors, the encyclopedia puts considerable emphasis on the idea of wellness. It discusses measures an individual can take to prevent illness and provides information about healthy lifestyle choices.

The *Macmillan Health Encyclopedia* is organized topically. Each of the nine volumes relates to an area covered in the school health curriculum. The encyclopedia also supplements course work in biology, psychology, home economics, and physical education. The volumes are organized as follows: 1. *Body Systems: Anatomy and Physiology*; 2. *Communicable Diseases: Symptoms, Diagnosis, Treatment*; 3. *Noncommunicable Diseases and Disorders: Symptoms, Diagnosis, Treatment*; 4. *Nutrition and Fitness*; 5. *Emotional and Mental Health*; 6. *Sexuality and Reproduction*; 7. *Drugs, Alcohol, and Tobacco*; 8. *Safety and Environmental Health*; 9. *Health-Care Systems/Cumulative Index*.

The information in the *Macmillan Health Encyclopedia* is clearly presented and easy to find. Entries are arranged in alphabetical order within each volume. An extensive system of cross-referencing directs the reader from a synonym to the main entry (GERMAN MEASLES see RUBELLA) and from one entry to additional information in other entries. Words printed in SMALL CAPITALS ("These substances, found in a number of NONPRESCRIPTION DRUGS . . .") indicate that there is an entry of that name in the volume. Most entries end with a list of "see also" cross-references to related topics. Entries within the same volume have no number (See also ANTI-INFLAMMATORY DRUGS); entries located in another volume include the volume number (See also HYPERTENSION, 3). All topics covered in a volume can be found in the index at the back of the book. There is also a comprehensive index to the set in Volume 9.

The extensive use of illustration includes colorful drawings, photographs, charts, and graphs to supplement and enrich the information presented in the text.

Questions of particular concern to the reader—When should I see a doctor? What are the risk factors? What can I do to prevent an illness?—are indicated by the following marginal notations: Consult a Physician, Risk Factors, and Healthy Choices.

Although difficult terms are explained within the context of the entry, each volume of the encyclopedia also has its own GLOSSARY. Located in the front of the book, the glossary provides brief definitions of medical or technical terms with which the reader may not be familiar.

A SUPPLEMENTARY SOURCES section at the back of the book contains a listing of suggested reading material, as well as organizations from which additional information can be obtained.

GLOSSARY

body system A group of interconnected and interdependent organs that act together to perform a certain function; the digestive system and the reproductive system are two examples.

diagnosis The process by which a physician identifies a disease or disorder.

disease/disorder An abnormal change in the structure or functioning of an organ or system in the body that produces a set of symptoms. The change may be caused by infection, heredity, injury, environment, or lifestyle or by a combination of these.

euthanasia The act of allowing or causing a relatively easy or painless death for a person suffering from a terminal illness.

health The physical, mental, and social well-being of a person. Health is not just the absence of disease.

immune system A group of chemicals and cells (including white blood cells and antibodies) that protects the body from harmful substances, such as disease-causing microorganisms.

inpatient A patient who stays in a hospital or other health-care facility while under medical treatment.

internist A physician who specializes in internal medicine, the diagnosis and nonsurgical treatment of diseases and disorders.

life span The length of an individual life.

microorganism Any plant or animal so small that it can be seen only through a microscope.

otorhinolaryngologist A physician who specializes in the treatment of diseases of the ear, nose, and throat.

outpatient A patient who receives medical care at a hospital or other health-care facility on a day basis, without being admitted overnight.

pathogen A microorganism, such as a bacterium or a virus, that can cause disease.

preventive care Health care that emphasizes good diet, exercise, immunizations, and regular checkups as ways of avoiding health problems or diagnosing them earlier.

primary care Medical care a person receives from a general practitioner, internist, pediatrician, or family physician, who is generally the first physician to be consulted for illness or preventive care. A primary care physician may refer a patient to a specialist, or secondary care physician.

secondary care Medical care a person receives from a specialist. The person may or may not be referred by a primary care physician.

specialist A physician who receives advanced training in and devotes his or her practice to a particular branch of medicine. Examples are cardiologist, dermatologist, and ophthalmologist.

tendon A tough, flexible, fibrous cord that joins muscle to bone or muscle to muscle in the body.

terminally ill Having an illness that can be expected to cause death, usually within a known time.

vaccine Substance containing killed or weakened viruses or bacteria; it is administered to give a person active immunity to the disease caused by a specific virus or bacterium.

▶ ALTERNATIVE HEALTH CARE

Alternative health care refers to medical practices that have not been widely accepted by the medical establishment in the United States and other Western countries. Many people turn to alternative health care because they are dissatisfied with the medical establishment's emphasis on treatment and cures rather than on prevention and healthy living. Others find that certain alternative medical practices can relieve their pain and suffering after regular medical care has failed to do so.

Holistic Health Holistic medicine emphasizes prevention of disease and treatment of the whole person. Practitioners examine not only the patient's body but all the other factors that contribute to a person's health. Such factors include nutrition, heredity, mental and spiritual health, economic problems, living conditions, and family relationships.

Acupuncture The ancient Chinese practice of acupuncture involves inserting needles into parts of the body along so-called meridians, or channels of energy. When the needles are inserted and vibrated at specific points, they are believed to affect the lines of energy and restore the ailing organ to health. No one is sure exactly how acupuncture works, but it has been known to relieve some painful conditions such as arthritis. It has also been used successfully as an anesthetic in certain operations and to help treat depression and addictions.

Chiropractic Chiropractic is an approach to health care based on the belief that aligning or "adjusting" the spine enables the muscles and organs of the body to heal on their own. Chiropractic doctors have been successful in relieving the pain of certain muscle and joint disorders. There is no evidence, however, that chiropractic has any effect on other serious diseases, such as cancer or heart disease.

Homeopathy Individuals who practice homeopathy believe they can relieve the symptoms of disease by prescribing minute amounts of a substance, such as a drug, that would cause the same symptoms in a healthy person. Homeopathy is based on the theory that a small amount of the substance will build up the body's natural defenses against the illness. Vaccination works in a similar way, but there is no scientific evidence that homeopathic remedies are effective in treating any illnesses. (See also CHIROPRACTOR; ACUPUNCTURE, 3.)

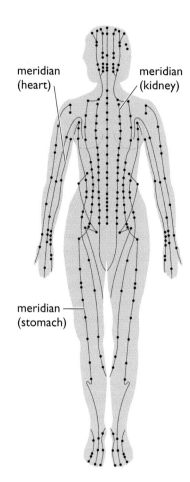

meridian (heart)

meridian (kidney)

meridian (stomach)

Acupuncture. *Acupuncture is based on the idea that there are channels of energy, called meridians, running through the body and that specific points along the meridians correspond to individual organs.*

▶ ANESTHESIOLOGIST

Anesthesiologists (AN us THEE zee AHL uh justs) are *physicians* who administer anesthetic drugs to patients to prevent pain during *surgery* and other medical procedures. They may give a *general anesthetic,* which makes the patient unconscious, or a *local anesthetic,* which controls pain in a specific area of the body. Anesthesiologists work with anesthetists—nurses or technicians who administer anesthetics under the supervision of an anesthesiologist.

Anesthesiologists and anesthetists are responsible for deciding which anesthetic drugs to use for each patient, determining the dosage,

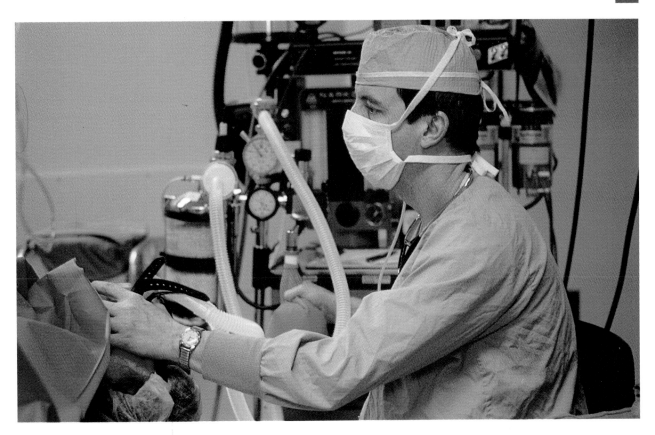

Administering Anesthetic Drugs. *Anesthesiologists and nurse anesthetists administer anesthetic drugs and monitor the patient throughout the medical procedure.*

and monitoring the patient's physical condition before, during, and after the procedure. They must also handle any medical emergencies arising from the use of anesthetic drugs.

Anesthesiologists must complete at least 2 years of special training after medical school to specialize in the field of anesthesiology. Nurse anesthetists must earn a degree in nursing, complete a 2-year training program in anesthesia, and pass a professional certification examination. (See also NURSING; PHYSICIANS (M.D.'s); ANESTHESIA, 3; ANESTHETIC DRUGS, 7.)

▶ **CARDIOLOGIST**   see PHYSICIANS (M.D.'s)

▶ **CENTERS FOR DISEASE CONTROL**   see DEPARTMENT OF HEALTH AND HUMAN SERVICES

▶ **CHIROPRACTOR**   A chiropractor is a health-care practitioner who treats pain and structural disorders by manipulating the muscles, joints, and spinal column. Chiropractors practice chiropractic medicine, a form of ALTERNATIVE HEALTH CARE that is based on the belief that using manipulation techniques

to make so-called adjustments to the spine promotes the healing of bodily ailments by improving the flow of nerve impulses to the brain. Chiropractors do not perform surgery or prescribe medication.

Chiropractic techniques can be useful in treating certain back problems and other joint and muscle disorders. Many chiropractors limit their practice to these problems, but some claim to treat a wide range of disorders. However, chiropractic has not been scientifically proved effective against illnesses such as heart disease, hypertension, and cancer.

A person interested in becoming a chiropractor must complete at least 2 years of college plus a 4-year program at a chiropractic college and pass a state licensing examination.

▶ CLINIC

A medical clinic usually provides primary (first-contact) care for people with injuries and illnesses. Some clinics are part of a hospital. Others are run by a group of doctors or community organizations. The staff of most clinics includes both general practitioners and specialists. Some clinics offer specific services such as prenatal care, mental health counseling, and drug treatment.

Clinics may be run by private, for-profit organizations or public, nonprofit organizations, some of which receive government funding. *Independent emergency centers,* or urgicenters, are private, for-profit clinics that offer drop-in care at any time of the day and often the night. These centers treat minor emergencies such as sprains, cuts, and other injuries.

Developments and Changes Before government funding of health care through Medicaid and Medicare, clinics attached to hospitals or OPDs (outpatient departments) offered free medical care to the poor. Medical students and residents (doctors in training) provided the

Urgicenters. *Independent emergency centers provide treatment for minor emergencies without an appointment.*

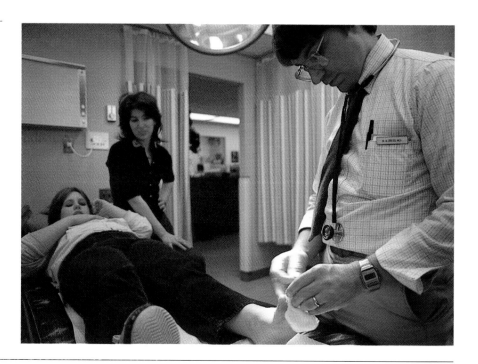

needed services under the supervision of experienced doctors. Today, government funding helps pay for some of those who cannot afford care. The use of clinics is expected to grow, especially in areas where services are scarce.

▶ **COUNSELOR**   **see PSYCHOTHERAPISTS**

▶ **DENTAL CARE**   Dental-care professionals help people care for their teeth and mouths and prevent, diagnose, and correct dental problems. Types of dental-care professionals include dentist, oral surgeon, orthodontist, and dental hygienist.

Dentist   A dentist is a doctor who is trained to recognize, treat, and prevent disorders of the teeth, gums, and jaws. Most dentists practice general dentistry: They clean teeth, fill cavities, extract teeth, and install crowns, bridges, and dentures. They also teach their patients how to prevent tooth disorders and gum disease.

A dentist in general practice must complete at least 2 years of college (although most complete 4) and a 4-year program at a dental college to earn a doctor of dental surgery (D.D.S.) degree or a doctor of dental medicine (D.M.D.) degree. A dentist must also pass a licensing examination in the state in which he or she intends to practice.

New dentists often work for an established dentist. Many then go into private practice by themselves or in association with other dentists. Most dentists employ dental hygienists and dental assistants.

Most people choose a dentist by asking family and friends for recommendations. General practitioners also refer their patients to specialists who treat difficult dental problems. In addition, local and state dental societies usually maintain reference services to help people find dentists and specialists.

When choosing a dentist, you should consider the dentist's education and experience. Also, look for a dentist who stresses disease prevention. Developing good oral hygiene can help you avoid problems with your teeth and gums in later years.

Oral Surgeon   An oral surgeon is a dental specialist who performs difficult tooth extractions and treats mouth and jaw injuries and malformations. Oral surgeons may remove impacted wisdom teeth, perform plastic surgery on the jaw or mouth, and fix a broken jaw. To become an oral surgeon, a person must obtain a degree in general dentistry, complete 4 years of specialized training, and pass a licensing examination.

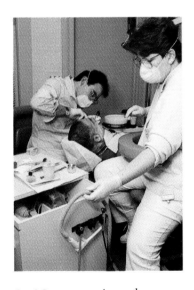

Oral Surgeon. *An oral surgeon performs difficult tooth extractions, such as when wisdom teeth become impacted, and treats mouth and jaw injuries, such as broken jaws.*

Orthodontist   An orthodontist specializes in realigning abnormally positioned teeth and improving the way the teeth in the upper and lower jaws fit together. This is usually done through the use of braces, which apply gentle pressure to move the teeth into the correct positions. Before affixing braces, orthodontists must sometimes remove certain

teeth to allow space for the teeth that are being moved. Orthodontists usually receive 4 years of specialized training in addition to a general dentistry degree. (See also ORTHODONTIC DEVICES, 3.)

Dental Hygienist Dental hygienists are licensed professionals who work for dentists. Their primary functions are to clean patients' teeth and teach patients how to care for their own teeth and gums. Some dental hygienists perform a variety of other tasks as well: They act as assistants to dentists by administering local anesthesia, keeping dental records, making appointments, performing preliminary examinations, and taking dental impressions and X rays.

To train to become a dental hygienist, a person must graduate from high school. Then he or she must complete a 2-year associate degree program or a 4-year bachelor's degree program in dental hygiene. All states require that dental hygienists be licensed to practice, and most states require that the hygienist pass a licensing test. (See also DENTAL EXAMINATION, 1; TOOTH, 1; DENTAL PROBLEMS, 3; DENTURES, 3; GUM DISEASE, 3.)

▷ DEPARTMENT OF HEALTH AND HUMAN SERVICES

The Department of Health and Human Services is a Cabinet-level department of the United States government that deals with public health, social welfare, and income security. Its four principal operating divisions are the Public Health Service, which provides the health-related services described below; the Health Care Financing Administration, which administers MEDICARE AND MEDICAID programs for elderly, disabled, and lower-income Americans; the Office of Human Development Services, which oversees programs for groups with special needs, such as children, the handicapped, and the aged; and the Social Security Administration, which administers federal social insurance programs.

The division most directly concerned with protecting and improving health is the Public Health Service, which consists of the following five agencies.

Food and Drug Administration The Food and Drug Administration (FDA) enforces laws that regulate the food, drug, and cosmetics industries. Through regulations, inspections, and testing procedures, the FDA tries to ensure that food, drug, and cosmetic products are pure, safe, and effective. The FDA also sets standards for truthful labeling on these products and monitors their production and shipment. (See also FOOD AND DRUG ADMINISTRATION, 7.)

> Through regulations, inspections, and testing procedures, the FDA tries to ensure that food, drug, and cosmetic products are pure, safe, and effective.

Centers for Disease Control The Centers for Disease Control (CDC) are a group of seven separate centers charged with preventing and controlling the spread of disease. The work of the centers includes conducting research on specific diseases, identifying and studying health problems internationally, and devising guidelines and overseeing programs for improved health. Two important aspects of this are immunization programs and efforts to track and analyze epidemics like AIDS.

Many CDC projects rely on medical data collected by the National Center for Health Statistics, one of the seven centers. The other centers

THE CDC AND NIH

Centers for Disease Control

National Center for Chronic Disease Prevention and Health Promotion

National Center for Environmental Health

National Center for Health Statistics

National Center for Infectious Diseases

National Center for Injury Prevention and Control

National Center for Prevention Services

National Institute for Occupational Safety and Health

National Institutes of Health

National Institute on Aging

National Institute of Allergy and Infectious Diseases

National Institute of Arthritis and Musculoskeletal and Skin Diseases

National Cancer Institute

National Institute of Child Health and Human Development

National Institute on Deafness and Other Communication Disorders

National Institute of Dental Research

National Institute of Diabetes and Digestive and Kidney Diseases

National Institute of Environmental Health Sciences

National Eye Institute

National Institute of General Medical Sciences

National Heart, Lung, and Blood Institute

National Institute of Neurological Disorders and Stroke

focus on areas such as infectious disease, lifestyle risks and chronic disease, and environmental health.

National Institutes of Health   The National Institutes of Health (NIH) comprise an agency whose main task is researching the causes and cures of diseases. Each of the 13 institutes focuses on a major disease or area of health. Examples include the National Cancer Institute and the National Heart, Lung, and Blood Institute. Other institutes study aging, allergies, dental disease, environmental diseases, children's health, and other health topics. The NIH also includes the Clinical Center, a research hospital that serves the institutes, and the National Library of Medicine, which is the largest medical library in the world. The international arm of the NIH is the Fogarty International Center. It conducts worldwide health research and helps other nations deal with their health problems.

Health Resources and Services Administration   The Health Resources and Services Administration supervises community health, family planning services, and health programs for mothers and children. It focuses on improving these services to individuals in areas without adequate health care. This agency also conducts research and supports programs that provide education and training for health workers.

Substance Abuse and Mental Health Services Administration
The Substance Abuse and Mental Health Services Administration oversees efforts to prevent alcoholism, drug addiction, and mental illness. One of its goals is to improve the treatment and rehabilitation of those affected by these diseases. (See also PREVENTIVE MEDICINE.)

▶ # DERMATOLOGIST   see PHYSICIANS (M.D.'s)

▶ # DIETITIAN   see NUTRITIONIST

▶ # EMERGENCY MEDICAL TECHNICIAN   An emergency medical technician (EMT) is a person who is trained to provide immediate assistance to people who are ill or injured in accidents until they can be seen by a physician. The capabilities of an EMT depend on the level of certification achieved. The four levels are nonambulance, ambulance, intermediate, and paramedic.

All levels of EMT are trained to perform cardiopulmonary resuscitation (CPR), deliver babies, and provide first aid treatment for wounds, broken bones, and shock. In addition to this basic training, an *EMT-ambulance* is certified to drive and maintain an ambulance. An *EMT-intermediate* is certified to provide more advanced types of medical care, such as assessing trauma and opening breathing passages. And an *EMT-paramedic*, the

EMT-Paramedic. *An EMT-paramedic is trained to provide advanced first aid, including giving intravenous fluids.*

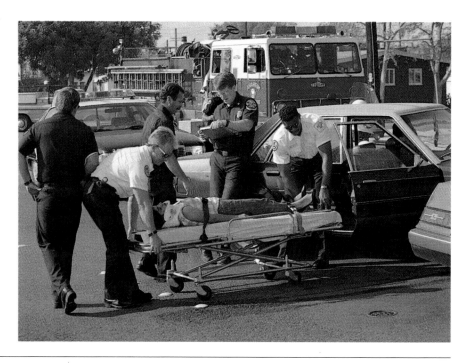

highest level, is certified to give medication and intravenous fluids and use technologically advanced machines like defibrillators, which can restart a stopped heart with an electric shock.

Standards vary, but most states require a person interested in becoming an EMT to complete a basic course of 110 hours of classroom training plus a 6-month internship in ambulance rescue work. Paramedics must take additional classes and pass a written and practical examination, which can take up to a year. Because they must work under conditions that can be emotionally and physically demanding, EMTs must be physically fit, have good judgment, and be able to act effectively during emergencies.

▶ EYE CARE

People in the eye-care field diagnose, treat, and correct eye and vision problems. Types of eye-care professionals include ophthalmologist, optometrist, and optician.

Ophthalmologist An ophthalmologist (AHF thuh MAHL uh just) is a medical doctor who specializes in the care of the eye. Ophthalmologists diagnose vision problems and treat them by prescribing glasses, contact lenses, and medications as well as performing eye surgery. Because they have medical training, ophthalmologists can often identify diseases or problems elsewhere in the body that may affect vision. Such diseases include diabetes, brain tumors, and multiple sclerosis. Ophthalmologists usually work closely with other medical doctors when treating a patient with one of these diseases.

Because the parts of the eye are so small, ophthalmologists often use microscopes and magnifying lenses when performing surgical procedures.

Ophthalmologists complete 4 years of college and 4 years of medical school before training an additional 3 years to specialize in ophthalmology. (See also PHYSICIANS (M.D.'s).)

Optometrist An optometrist is a specialist who examines your eyes and, if necessary, prescribes and fits glasses or contact lenses. Optometrists may also suggest eye exercises to correct certain vision problems. Eye examinations measure your ability to see things nearby and at a distance. They also determine how well your eyes work together, in reading and other activities. Optometrists are not medical doctors; therefore, they refer patients who require prescription medication or surgery to an ophthalmologist.

In the United States, a license is required to practice optometry. An optometrist must attend at least 2 years of college and complete 4 years of optometry school to earn a doctor of optometry (O.D.) degree. After graduating from optometry school, optometrists must pass a state examination to obtain a license to practice.

Optician An optician fills doctors' prescriptions for glasses and contact lenses. Some opticians actually make the glasses by grinding the glass and fitting the lenses into the frames. Other opticians help people choose frames that suit them. After the glasses have been made, these

> Eye examinations measure your ability to see things nearby and at a distance. They also determine how well your eyes work together.

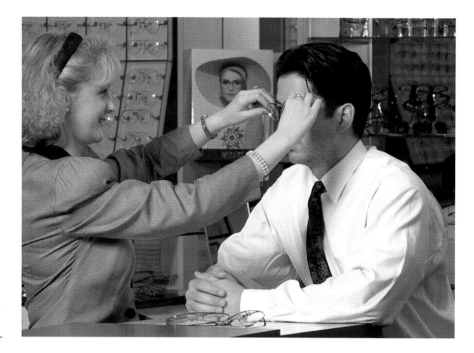

Optician. *Opticians are eye-care professionals who fill prescriptions for glasses and contact lenses.*

opticians measure and adjust the glasses for the proper fit. Opticians do not have the training required to perform eye examinations or to write prescriptions.

Most opticians work either in a store that sells glasses and contact lenses or in a laboratory that makes them. Some opticians work for optometrists or ophthalmologists.

To become an optician, a person should have a high school diploma. Opticians are usually trained for several years on the job. A person may also take a 2-year college program to get training. Opticians must be licensed to practice in some states. (See also EYE DISORDERS, **3**; EYE TEST, **3**; VISION PROBLEMS, **3**.)

▶ GENETIC COUNSELOR

RISK FACTORS
▶ ▶ ▶ ▶ ▶ ▶

Genetic counselors are health-care professionals, usually *physicians* with training in genetics, who counsel couples at risk of producing a child with an inherited disorder such as Down syndrome, spina bifida, or Tay-Sachs disease. They provide information about genetic disorders, assess the risk of producing a child with a disorder, and perform various tests to detect the presence of a disorder. Older couples, couples who have a history of genetic diseases or birth defects in their families, and couples who have already had a child with an inherited disorder are frequently referred to genetic counselors.

The genetic counselor takes a complete family medical history of both parents to assess the likelihood that their offspring will be born with an inherited disease. The counselor may also perform diagnostic tests like amniocentesis on the fetus or chromosome tests on the parents and any other offspring to determine whether certain abnormalities are present. (See also PHYSICIANS (M.D.'s); GENETICS, **6**; GENETIC SCREENING, **6**.)

▶ GERONTOLOGIST

A gerontologist studies the process of aging and often works with the elderly. Gerontologists examine aging from many perspectives. They consider the developmental, biological, medical, sociological, and psychological aspects of aging. The medical specialty that treats the elderly is called *geriatrics*.

Most gerontologists believe that aging begins when a person's physical growth stops and cells die faster than they reproduce (usually at approximately 25 years of age). Gerontologists measure age in three different ways. Chronological age is based on the number of years a person has lived. Biological age is determined by how fit a person's body is. And social age compares a person's behavior with standards of behavior expected of someone at that particular chronological age.

▶ GROUP MEDICAL CARE

In group medical care or group practice, more than two physicians share office space, equipment, and staff. The single-specialty group practice offers only one type of medical care, such as pediatrics (care of children). You may see any member of the group when you visit because each provides the same type of services. The multispecialty group practice offers several types of specialists working together. You may need to see a cardiologist for your heart, a nutritionist for diet help, or a physical therapist for exercise advice.

One advantage of group medical care is that doctors can easily consult with and inform each other. Because they all are affected by the group's reputation, each checks on the performance of the others to maintain high-quality care. In addition, physicians in a group practice often organize their schedules so as to offer extended office hours and on-call services. (See also CLINIC; PHYSICIANS (M.D.'s).)

▶ GYNECOLOGIST   see PHYSICIANS (M.D.'s)

▶ HEALTH-CARE SYSTEM

A health-care system consists of all the medical care that is available to the people of a nation, the way that medical care is delivered, and the way it is paid for. The American health-care system boasts the world's most advanced technology and many of the best-trained doctors, dentists, and nurses. However, it is also the most expensive system in the world, which places the best medical care out of the reach of millions of Americans.

Medical Care   In the United States, there are nearly two doctors for every thousand people. The availability of medical care is uneven, however, because physicians tend to set up practices in or near big cities, leaving many small towns and rural areas with limited health care. Years

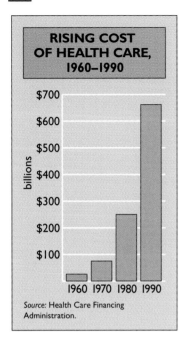

RISING COST OF HEALTH CARE, 1960–1990

billions

$700
$600
$500
$400
$300
$200
$100

1960 1970 1980 1990

Source: Health Care Financing Administration.

ago, most physicians practiced alone, but today many practice in groups. Vast increases in medical knowledge and complicated technologies have also led the majority of physicians to become specialists in limited areas of medicine. General practitioners and family doctors are in demand.

Technological advances, such as organ transplants, laser surgery, CAT (computerized axial tomography) scans, and genetic engineering to create new medicines, help save many lives by making it possible to detect and treat many diseases and disorders that once were untreatable. Yet the costs of these technologies are raising the costs of hospital stays, tests, surgeries, and other medical procedures (see graph: Rising Cost of Health Care, 1960–1990).

Paying for Medical Care In the United States, a majority of medical costs are paid by insurance companies. In the past, many corporations and businesses provided their employees with health-insurance programs that paid all or most medical costs. Because the cost of health care has skyrocketed, however, more and more businesses are finding that they cannot afford the bill for complete health-care coverage. Indeed, a large number of small businesses cannot afford to provide HEALTH INSURANCE at all.

Millions of Americans pay for their own health insurance by joining group plans in which the members share the costs of medical care. In addition, the federal and state governments provide health insurance for people older than the age of 65 (*Medicare*) and for the very poor (*Medicaid*). Despite these options, an estimated 40 million Americans are not poor enough to qualify for government health insurance but are too poor to buy their own insurance. Typically, they request medical care only in dire emergencies. (See also MEDICARE AND MEDICAID.)

Other Health-Care System Models In a number of other countries, including Canada and Great Britain, the government funds and organizes health care for its citizens. This system is often called *socialized medicine.* Although the systems vary from country to country, in most cases doctors and other health-care workers are paid by the government. Government-supported health care does have drawbacks, however. Patients generally have fewer choices about which physicians they can see and what medical services they can receive, and they often have to wait some time for nonemergency procedures and surgery. (See also CLINIC; HEALTH MAINTENANCE ORGANIZATION.)

▶ **HEALTH-CARE WORKERS** Many people besides medical doctors and nurses help you care for your health. These health-care workers include practitioners, technicians, therapists, personal-care workers, and medical assistants.

Practitioners Practitioners are qualified to provide many of the same kinds of services as medical doctors. They are specially trained in one area, such as emergency treatment or dental hygiene. The *optometrist* who tests people's vision and prescribes eyeglasses is a practitioner, as is a *midwife* who cares for pregnant women and delivers babies. (See also EMERGENCY MEDICAL TECHNICIAN; EYE CARE; NURSING; PODIATRIST.)

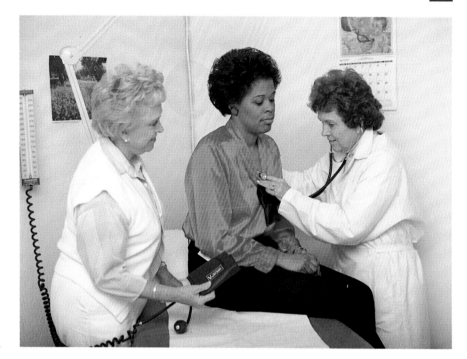

Medical Assistants. *Medical assistants play an important role in doctors' offices and clinics. Their duties may include scheduling and receiving patients, handling billing, assisting physicians in examinations and treatments, and performing certain tests.*

Technicians   Technicians operate the many machines used in hospitals, doctors' offices, and laboratories to test and treat patients. They also perform tests, such as blood and urine analyses, that provide doctors with information about the health of a patient's body. Technicians often have special training in one area. For example, some work only with X rays and tests based on radiation. (See also MEDICAL TECHNOLOGISTS AND TECHNICIANS.)

Therapists   Therapists work with people to eliminate or improve specific health problems, often through a hands-on technique like exercise. Each is trained in a particular health field, such as the treatment of emotional difficulties or physical injuries. One kind of therapist helps someone overcome a lisp; another kind uses music and dance to help people who are depressed feel better. (See also OCCUPATIONAL THERAPIST; PHYSICAL THERAPIST; SPEECH THERAPY.)

Personal Health-Care Workers   Sometimes people become too sick or physically unable to perform personal tasks for themselves. Personal-care workers help such people eat, bathe, and get dressed either in the hospital or at home. (See also HOME HEALTH SERVICES.)

▶ **HEALTH EDUCATOR**   Health educators are concerned with lifestyle and behavior related to health. They design programs to teach people how to adopt healthier lifestyles and how to prevent or manage diseases. They are employed in schools, the health-care industry, businesses, and community settings.

Health educators in schools develop and teach classroom topics such as sex education, drugs and drug abuse, and disease prevention. In other sectors, health educators run programs to encourage people to quit

smoking or control their weight. They also plan health exhibits and health fairs and organize support groups for people with illnesses like heart or kidney disease and cancer.

Health-education careers are expected to grow in the future as government and industry become increasingly interested in promoting a healthier population. A health-education career requires a 4-year college degree in health education. Health educators in schools must usually be certified to teach.

▶ **HEALTH INSURANCE**   Health insurance is a means of ensuring that medical expenses can be paid. Most people do not know whether or when they will get sick, so they (or their employers) contribute a monthly payment, or premium, to an insurance plan. If an individual in the plan gets sick, the insurance company then pays part or all of the medical bills out of the pool of premium payments.

Types of Coverage   Insurance companies offer various types of coverage. *Basic health insurance* covers a portion of hospital, medical, and surgical expenses. *Major medical insurance* pays for larger medical expenses that can result from long or serious illnesses or injuries. This type of insurance is intended to supplement basic health insurance. *Disability insurance* pays an income to people who are not able to work because of illness or injury.

The costs of health care in the United States have been rising rapidly in recent years, and the cost of health insurance has soared. Many employers continue to provide health insurance to their workers as a job

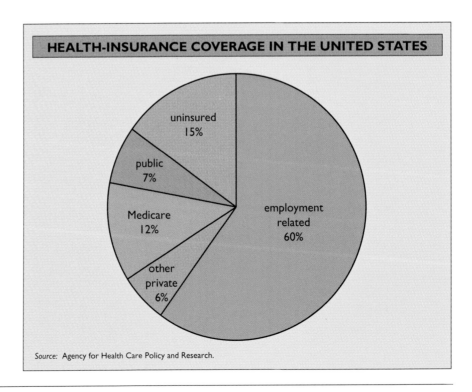

HEALTH-INSURANCE COVERAGE IN THE UNITED STATES

uninsured 15%
public 7%
Medicare 12%
other private 6%
employment related 60%

Source: Agency for Health Care Policy and Research.

benefit, but many can no longer afford to do so and are requiring their employees to carry a larger share of the cost. And the majority of people who have jobs with few benefits, or who are unemployed, cannot afford the high cost of individual insurance. As a result, an estimated 40 million Americans have no health insurance at all.

A National Health-Care Program   Today, health-care coverage is a pressing social issue. There has been much talk about a national health-care program that would regulate costs for medical procedures and provide broader access to health care through improved health-insurance plans. Many people recognize that changes to the current system are needed. So far, however, there is no agreement on just what the changes should be. (See also HEALTH-CARE SYSTEM; HEALTH MAINTENANCE ORGANIZATION; MEDICARE AND MEDICAID.)

▶ HEALTH MAINTENANCE ORGANIZATION   A health maintenance organization (HMO) offers individuals and families a variety of medical services for a prepaid annual or monthly membership fee. Members are assigned a primary physician and, in most cases, are restricted to specialists and hospitals that are approved by the HMO. HMO programs usually offer complete coverage regardless of whether members need a routine checkup or must be hospitalized for a serious illness.

HMO programs were developed during the 1930s to encourage the prevention of disease through checkups, screenings, and health education in order to reduce costs. During the 1970s, health-care bills soared. In response, the government and other organizations offered financial support to spur HMO growth. HMOs have succeeded in cutting costs mainly through fewer and shorter hospital stays as a result of early diagnosis and treatment. Today there are more than 400 HMOs serving nearly 20 million Americans.

You may join an HMO through your employer, union, or professional organization. Like any health-care plan, the HMO has its pros and cons. You may not be free to choose your own doctor, specialists, or hospital. On the other hand, an HMO usually offers more complete coverage than a regular insurance plan and gives you quick access. Before joining a health maintenance organization, find out about its membership policies. Make sure that the participating hospitals are accredited and that the physicians are board certified. Compare costs of HMO membership with those of an insurance policy that offers comparable coverage.

▶ HOME HEALTH SERVICES   Home health services are medical and nonmedical services provided to elderly and disabled people who are permanently housebound or to patients who have recently returned home from a hospital or nursing home. These services include nursing care, therapy, and

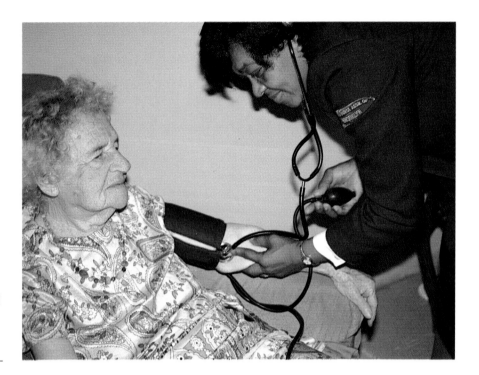

Visiting Nurse. *A visiting nurse can provide many medical services at home in order to allow patients to stay out of the hospital.*

housekeeping. They enable people who would otherwise have to stay in a hospital to remain at home and retain their independence.

Home health services include both skilled and supportive types of services. Skilled professional services are provided by *visiting nurses,* who give injections, change dressings, and monitor medications; physical, speech, and occupational therapists; and professionals in dental, nutritional, and laboratory services. Supportive services are provided by *home health aides,* who help with such tasks as bathing and grooming, housekeeping, changing bed linens, and shopping. Supportive services also include programs like Meals-on-Wheels, a nonprofit agency that delivers daily hot meals to elderly people who are unable to cook.

A hospital social worker can help patients determine what kind of home health care they need and can assist in choosing an agency. Some volunteer agencies also provide information or advice on home health care. These include the United Way, American Cancer Society, and Arthritis Foundation.

Home health services can be expensive, although part of the cost is usually covered by MEDICARE AND MEDICAID or private insurance plans. (See also HEALTH-CARE WORKERS; NURSING; OCCUPATIONAL THERAPIST; PHYSICAL THERAPIST.)

▶ **HOSPICE**

Hospice is a type of medical care for terminally ill patients and their families. Based on the special physical and emotional needs of the terminally ill, hospice care offers an alternative to traditional hospital care. Hospice programs may be located in a special section of a hospital, in a separate hospice facility, or in a dying person's home. Patients who are not expected

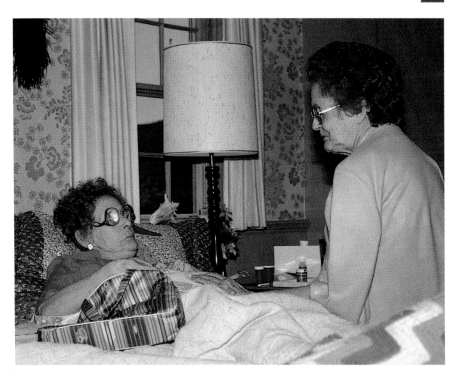

Hospice Care. *Hospice programs offer terminally ill patients an alternative to living out their final weeks or months in a hospital.*

to live more than 6 months may be admitted to a hospice program by their physician.

Characteristics of Hospice Care Hospice programs offer a team approach to care that involves the patients and their families, physicians, nurses, social workers, clergy, and volunteers. People who are terminally ill often have two main fears—pain and loneliness. Hospice programs try to deal with these concerns by providing a combination of medicine and pain-control techniques to keep the patient as comfortable as possible and also by offering emotional and spiritual support. A variety of community services are used to allow the patient to remain at home as long as possible. Hospice care does not include procedures or equipment such as respirators designed to lengthen a person's life.

Hospice care generally costs less than hospital care, and it has been included as a Medicare benefit since 1982. A growing number of private insurance companies provide hospice benefits as part of basic health coverage or as an option. (See also DYING AND BEREAVEMENT, **5.**)

▶ **HOSPITAL**

A hospital is a facility where doctors, nurses, and other health-care professionals care for seriously ill patients, administer complicated tests and medical procedures, and perform surgery.

Some hospitals are owned by private, profit-making corporations; others are owned by the communities in which they are located or by other nonprofit organizations such as churches and service clubs. The federal and state governments also operate many hospitals. Some hospitals specialize in caring only for certain kinds of patients, such as children, the

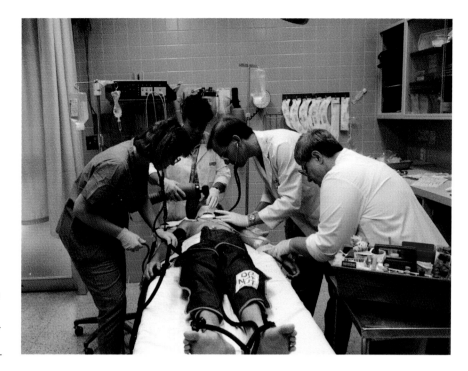

Emergency Department. *The physicians, nurses, and paramedics working in the emergency department of a hospital care for people in need of immediate medical attention.*

mentally ill, or military veterans. Others are teaching hospitals where medical and nursing students receive on-the-job training.

History   The first hospitals were founded by Buddhist monks in India in the third century B.C. In the Middle Ages, Christian religious orders established hospitals in cities throughout Europe. The first hospital in the United States was built by the Dutch in 1658 in what is now New York City. For centuries, hospitals were places that treated people who were too poor to be cared for at home. The reputation of hospitals suffered from a high mortality rate until the 1800s, when scientists discovered *anesthetics* to kill pain and developed a system of *antisepsis*, the killing of germs, to prevent the spread of disease.

The Modern Hospital   The typical hospital today is separated into several departments that carry out various functions. The *emergency department* (or emergency room) cares for people in need of immediate medical attention, such as those who have had a heart attack or received a gunshot wound. This department may also treat people who do not have their own family doctors. The *intensive care unit* provides nearly one-on-one nursing care and high-tech monitoring for gravely ill patients. *Coronary care units* are similar to intensive care units except that they treat only patients who have had heart attacks or related diseases. Most hospitals have large *radiology departments* that perform many kinds of diagnostic tests, including *X-ray examinations*.

In recent years, many hospitals have established or expanded *outpatient departments* to care for patients who need to come to the hospital for tests or therapy but who are not sick enough to be hospitalized. Similarly, many hospitals also have ambulatory (or outpatient) surgery departments that perform minor surgical procedures on patients who do not need to be kept in the hospital overnight. (See also CLINIC; HOSPICE; NURSING HOME; REHABILITATION CENTER.)

▶ **INTERNIST**   see PHYSICIANS (M.D.'s)

▶ **LICENSED PRACTICAL NURSE**   see NURSING

▶ **MARRIAGE COUNSELOR**   see PSYCHOTHERAPISTS

▶ **MEDICAL ETHICS**   Medical ethics (also called bioethics) is a rapidly growing field of study that deals with the difficult issues involved in decisions about patient care. Enormous technological advances now enable physicians to make use of life-support equipment, abortion, medical research and testing, and organ transplants. But in many cases, questions arise about the consequences of these capabilities and about who should make decisions regarding their use—the patient, the doctor, the patient's family, or all three.

Life Support   One of the earliest medical-ethics issues to gain public attention involved withdrawing life-support equipment from permanently unconscious (comatose) patients. Physicians have long recognized the right of patients to make decisions about their care, but who should make the decision when the patient is comatose? In 1976, the New Jersey Supreme Court ruled that the family of Karen Ann Quinlan, a permanently comatose young woman, had the right to ask that her respirator be turned off. The decision was a landmark in legal and medical history because it gave family members the right to decide for an incompetent patient.

Since the Quinlan case, many other issues of medical ethics have been raised about death and dying. Many states now have *right-to-die* laws granting terminally ill patients the right to refuse medical treatment that will prolong their lives. Many people now draw up *living wills*, documents in which they give instructions about the use of life-sustaining medical treatment. Some individuals have performed *euthanasia* on terminally ill people, that is, have assisted them in taking their own lives. This active assistance, often called mercy killing, is against the law in all states. Most doctors oppose euthanasia on the grounds that a physician's duty is to save lives no matter what the circumstances.

Birth   Many medical-ethics issues are concerned with birth. One of the most controversial concerns abortion. In 1973, the U.S. Supreme Court ruled that women have a Constitutional right to have an abortion. Since then, antiabortion (also called *pro-life*) activists have worked to have the ruling overturned, and *pro-choice* activists have worked to maintain it. In 1992, the Supreme Court upheld a woman's right to abortion but allowed states to impose certain limitations.

Other issues involve *in vitro fertilization,* the fertilizing of a woman's egg in a laboratory dish, and *surrogate mothers,* women who carry an infertile couple's fetus for them. One case involving a surrogate mother concerned whether the woman had the right to keep the child herself after agreeing to carry it for another couple.

Medical Research and Testing   Research into new medical treatments and drugs raises a host of bioethical concerns. A great deal of medical research involves *animal research.* Animal-rights activists want to ban research that subjects animals to painful or lethal experiments. Research on humans raises other troubling questions. All experimental procedures and drug testing must be carried out on humans as well as on animals. The primary ethical requirement in all human research is that the people involved be given complete, detailed information about the experiment so that they can make an informed decision about whether to participate. *Genetic engineering,* the manipulation of genes to cure diseases and create new drugs and foods, is a subject that makes many people uneasy. They are concerned about whether this new technology is safe and morally justified.

Transplants   One important technological advance, *organ transplants,* raises questions about who should receive scarce donor organs. Most medical centers that perform transplants have developed strict guidelines designed to ensure that organs go to people who can benefit the most from them.

New technology and the allocation of scarce resources will continue to create new dilemmas and controversies. In some cases, the decisions are easy to make. In others, they are agonizing. Most large medical centers have created ethics committees to help doctors, patients, and their families make difficult decisions. These committees usually include physicians, nurses, administrators, lawyers, and lay people who bring different experiences and perspectives to the decision-making process. (See also TRANSPLANT SURGERY, 3; ABORTION, 6; CLINICAL DRUG TRIALS, 7; GENETIC ENGINEERING, 8.)

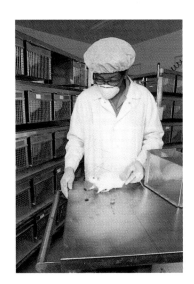

Animal Research.   *Using animals for medical testing is a controversial ethical issue.*

▶ **MEDICAL INSURANCE**   **see** HEALTH INSURANCE

▶ **MEDICAL TECHNOLOGISTS AND TECHNICIANS**   Medical technologists and technicians are health-care workers who perform laboratory tests and operate sophisticated medical equipment to help doctors diagnose and treat diseases. They work in hospitals, laboratories, doctors' offices, research institutes, and colleges and universities and perform many complex and routine procedures under the supervision of *physicians.*

Technologists and technicians specialize in one of several areas. *Medical laboratory technologists* conduct complicated chemical tests on body tissues and fluids. *Medical laboratory technicians* perform laboratory

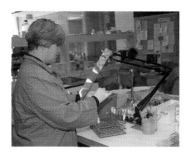

Medical Laboratory Technologists. *Laboratory technologists perform complicated tests on samples of body tissues and fluids.*

tests on tissues and body fluids under the supervision of a medical laboratory technologist. *Cytotechnologists* prepare cell samples for microscopic examinations, such as those to detect cancer. *Nuclear medicine technologists* use radioactive substances and radiation-detecting devices to diagnose disease. *Radiologic technologists* use X-ray examinations and other imaging devices to diagnose and treat disease. *Surgical technologists* prepare operating rooms and equipment for surgery.

Generally, a medical technician is less highly trained than a technologist and is responsible for less complicated procedures. A medical technician must graduate from high school and complete a 1- to 2-year course at a community college, technical school, or hospital. Technologists typically must complete a 4-year training course. (See also ANESTHESIOLOGIST; PHYSICIANS (M.D.'s); RADIOLOGIST; SURGEON.)

▶ MEDICARE AND MEDICAID

Medicare and Medicaid are government HEALTH INSURANCE programs. Medicare is a federal program that provides health-care coverage primarily for senior citizens and people who are disabled. Medicaid, administered by state governments under federal guidelines, provides coverage for people of any age who are poor.

Medicare The Medicare program has two parts. *Medicare A* covers a portion of medically necessary hospitalization expenses, as well as skilled nursing care, home health care, or hospice care. Under Medicare A, there is a yearly deductible amount that the patient must pay for hospitalization; in addition, if the illness lasts more than 2 months, the patient must pay a portion of the costs. All eligible Americans receive Medicare A. *Medicare B* is an optional plan intended to supplement the benefits provided by Medicare A. It covers physicians' and surgeons' fees and other health-care services, including tests, outpatient services, and certain medical supplies. Medicare B requires payment of a monthly premium.

Medicaid Medicaid programs vary considerably from state to state. In general, Medicaid covers all or part of hospitalization and medical expenses for people who receive or are eligible for other types of welfare assistance. Over recent years, limited availability of public funds combined with skyrocketing health-care costs have caused some states to tighten eligibility requirements or limit the range of coverage. (See also HEALTH-CARE SYSTEM.)

▶ MIDWIFE   see NURSING

▶ NATIONAL INSTITUTES OF HEALTH   see DEPARTMENT OF HEALTH AND HUMAN SERVICES

▷ **NURSING**

Nurses are people who provide care for patients under the direction of a physician and help people care for their health. Types of nurses include registered nurse (R.N.), licensed practical nurse (L.P.N.), and nurses' aide or nursing assistant.

Registered Nurse   A registered nurse is a person who has completed a nursing program that combines academic and practical training, has received a degree or diploma, and has passed a state licensing examination. People who wish to become registered nurses can get their training in one of several ways. Some community colleges offer a 2-year associate degree program. Others provide training in a 4-year bachelor's degree program. Certain hospitals conduct a 3-year training course. Students who complete this program receive a diploma.

The majority of registered nurses work in hospitals. Others work in NURSING HOMES or rehabilitation centers. Some work in clinics or in doctors' offices. Still others care for patients in their homes.

There are several kinds of R.N.'s. For example, general duty nurses are responsible for the care of a number of patients who may have different medical problems and needs. These R.N.'s monitor patient progress, oversee the keeping of patient records, give medications, and supervise personal-care providers, nurses' aides, and practical nurses.

Some R.N.'s complete additional training (usually a master's degree) and specialize in a particular area, such as those who become nurse practitioners and nurse midwives. A *nurse practitioner* performs many of the duties of a doctor, including giving physical examinations and treating patients. Nurse practitioners are not allowed to prescribe medicine, however, and they are generally under the supervision of a physician. A *nurse midwife* assists pregnant women before and during delivery and may also help with the care of newborns. To become a nurse midwife, a person must meet the graduate training standards of the American College of Nurse-Midwives. Nurse midwives are licensed and often work with an obstetrician. Other R.N.'s become *nurse anesthetists* and operating room nurses. (See also ANESTHESIOLOGIST.)

Nursing.   *The nursing field offers a range of duties, depending on training. Nurses' aides (left) perform basic patient-care tasks. Nurse practitioners (right) are qualified to perform physical examinations.*

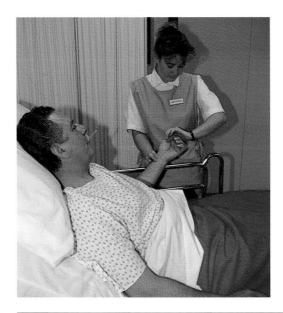

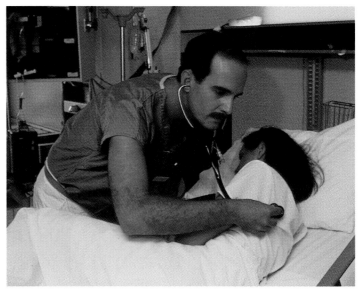

Licensed Practical Nurse   A licensed practical nurse, also known as a licensed vocational nurse (L.V.N.) in some areas, assists a doctor or registered nurse in caring for patients. L.P.N.'s help carry out doctors' treatment plans by checking patients' blood pressure and temperature, putting on bandages, and providing other routine care. They also monitor and report patient progress to doctors and other members of the health-care team. In addition, these nurses may directly supervise nurses' aides.

Prospective L.P.N.'s train for 2 years, both in the classroom and in a medical setting with real patients. Then they must pass a state test to become licensed. Licensed practical nurses work in doctors' offices, hospitals, and nursing homes, as well as in business organizations, schools, and private homes.

Nurses' Aide   A nurses' aide, or nursing assistant, performs basic tasks, such as feeding and bathing patients, in a hospital or other health-care facility under the supervision of R.N.'s and L.P.N.'s. Nurses' aides may or may not have a formal education in nursing. However, nurses' aides who work in nursing homes must pass a training course and pass a state certification examination. (See also HEALTH-CARE WORKERS; HOME HEALTH SERVICES; PHYSICIANS (M.D.'s); SURGEON.)

▶ NURSING HOME
A nursing home is a facility that provides its residents with some level of medical and personal care in addition to food and lodging. Most residents are elderly people who can no longer manage at home. As the number of older Americans grows, so does the number of nursing homes. Most of these are privately run for profit; the rest are operated by volunteer organizations or the government. Some nursing homes are licensed by state or local agencies. The amount of health care provided differs in the three main types of nursing homes.

> Most nursing home residents are elderly people who can no longer manage at home. As the number of older Americans grows, so does the number of nursing homes.

Types of Nursing Homes   *Residential-Care Facilities* (RCFs) offer a limited amount of health care. For example, the staff will make sure that residents take their medication correctly. Equally important, RCF residents gain the security of knowing that they are not alone. At an *Intermediate-Care Facility* (ICF), some nursing care is provided, and programs such as physical or speech therapy may be offered. Some ICFs also offer residents a sense of community through organized social activities. The greatest amount of health care can be found at *Skilled Nursing Facilities* (SNFs). These provide 24-hour nursing care, and many have a doctor on staff.

Paying for Nursing Home Care   Nursing home care is very expensive and usually not paid for by insurance. Medicare, government health insurance for people older than the age of 65, pays just for the first several months. After that, if a person cannot pay for his or her care, another government program called Medicaid takes over. Medicare or Medicaid pays only for care in intermediate-care and skilled nursing facilities, however, not in residential-care facilities. (See also MEDICARE AND MEDICAID; NURSING; REHABILITATION CENTER.)

▶ NUTRITIONIST

Nutritionists are people who are trained in the science of nutrition and who apply that training in a variety of settings. Some nutritionists provide private counseling to individuals who need dietary advice. Some guide food manufacturers in the preparation of healthful meals. And many work in hospitals and institutions. Depending on the training they receive, and the type of work they do, nutritionists may be called *dietitians*.

There are different types of dietitians. *Administrative dietitians* plan meals for groups of people in institutions such as schools, nursing homes, industrial plants, and prisons. They must pay attention not only to the nutritional content of the meals, but also to the cost and preparation. *Clinical dietitians* plan meals and diets for people with special needs. These people may include hospital patients; people with diabetes, cancer, allergies, hypertension, or heart disease; and people who are overweight or underweight. A clinical dietitian's work involves devising a diet that meets nutritional needs and teaching a person how to choose and prepare special foods.

The roles of nutritionists and dietitians have expanded as Americans have become more interested in healthful eating. Today, nutritionists are involved in athletic and fitness programs, in summer camps for children with weight problems, and in a variety of public health programs.

A person interested in becoming a nutritionist must major in nutrition or food-service management in college and complete additional training approved by the American Dietetic Association (ADA). He or she must also pass a test given by the ADA to become a *registered dietitian* (RD), a qualification that is usually required for work in a hospital or institution. (See also NUTRITION, **4.**)

▶ OBSTETRICIAN   see PHYSICIANS (M.D.'s)

▶ OCCUPATIONAL THERAPIST

Occupational therapists are professional HEALTH-CARE WORKERS who help patients overcome physical and emotional disabilities that may result from an accident, illness, aging, or psychological problems. The goal of occupational therapy is for patients to regain the ability to live and work as independently as possible.

An occupational therapist uses various activities to help patients regain use of muscles and develop skills. The therapy may involve simple exercises or games or the use of activities such as knitting or painting, which provide both physical and mental stimulation. The activities used and the goals of therapy depend on the individual case. Some patients need to learn new ways to perform simple daily activities, such as dressing, eating, and cooking. Others benefit from learning new skills that may be useful for employment.

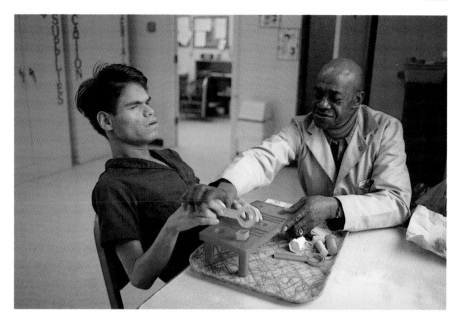

Occupational Therapy. *Occupational therapy helps people disabled by physical or emotional problems to regain their independence.*

Occupational therapists must have either a bachelor's degree in occupational therapy or a 1- to 2-year course in occupational therapy following an undergraduate degree in another area. In most states it is necessary to pass a qualifying examination to be licensed to practice. (See also HOME HEALTH SERVICES; PHYSICAL THERAPIST.)

▶ **ONCOLOGIST** see PHYSICIANS (M.D.'s)

▶ **OPHTHALMOLOGIST** see EYE CARE

▶ **OPTOMETRIST** see EYE CARE

▶ **ORTHOPEDIST** see PHYSICIANS (M.D.'s)

▶ **OSTEOPATHIC PHYSICIANS (D.O.'S)** Osteopathic physicians, or Doctors of Osteopathy (D.O.'s), are one of two types of medical doctors in the United States. Like the other type, Doctors of Medicine (M.D.'s), osteopathic physicians are fully trained and qualified to perform surgery, prescribe medication, and practice in all areas of medicine. The main

difference between D.O.'s and M.D.'s is in the philosophy of medicine rather than in the level of training or skill.

Osteopathic physicians practice a system of health care called osteopathy. *Osteopathy* is based on the idea that the systems of the body work in unison, each one influencing the function of others and of the entire body. In the osteopathic philosophy, the musculoskeletal system—the spinal column, bones, muscles, nerves, and tendons—plays a particularly important role in the body's health. Osteopathic physicians believe in emphasizing prevention, fitness, and the body's ability to heal itself.

In addition to traditional methods of diagnosing and treating disease, osteopathic physicians use a technique called *osteopathic manipulative treatment* (OMT). With OMT, physicians use their hands to check and realign the musculoskeletal system, believing that this promotes the body's natural tendency toward health.

A person interested in becoming an osteopathic physician must complete 4 years of college and 4 years of training at an osteopathic medical school. This is usually followed by a year of internship and 1 to 5 years of training in a chosen specialty at an osteopathic hospital. (See also ALTERNATIVE HEALTH CARE; PHYSICIANS (M.D.'S).)

▶ **PARAMEDIC**   **see EMERGENCY MEDICAL TECHNICIAN**

▶ **PATHOLOGIST**   A pathologist is a *physician* who investigates changes in the tissues and organs of the body that are caused by disease. Pathologists do not treat patients directly but often work closely with the physicians who do.

Laboratory tests performed by pathologists include examinations of the blood, urine, organs, and tissues. These tests are used to diagnose and determine the extent of disease. Pathologists also study diseased tissue

Pathologist. *Pathologists study tissue samples to diagnose and determine the extent of a disease.*

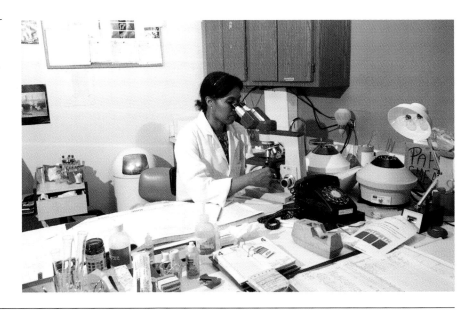

and body parts removed during surgery. In addition, when the reason for a patient's death is unclear, a pathologist may perform a special examination of the corpse, known as an *autopsy,* to determine the cause of a person's death or, in some cases, to learn more about a disease or disorder.

Pathologists must complete college and 4 years of medical school, plus 3 or more years as a resident in the field of pathology. Many pathologists go on to acquire additional expertise in a subspecialty of pathology, such as *hematology* (the study of blood and its diseases). (See also PHYSICIANS (M.D.'s); AUTOPSY, **2.**)

▶ PATIENTS' RIGHTS

Patients' rights are the legal rights and ethical principles that empower medical consumers (patients) to participate in their own medical care. The American Hospital Association first published a Patients' Bill of Rights in 1973. It is primarily a list of objectives that health-care workers are expected to meet in dealing with patients.

The most important right that patients possess is the right to *informed consent.* Informed consent means that patients must be completely informed about a proposed medical treatment and must consent to that treatment. Patients must be told of the risks and benefits of the treatment as well as information on alternative treatments in clear, understandable language.

As medical technology has advanced, the right to refuse treatment has become important to many individuals. This right can conflict, however, with the duty of physicians to make full use of their training and available resources to save lives. In most states, people can sign "living wills" to protect this right. Living wills instruct physicians to withhold or discontinue care that would only prolong suffering in the terminal phase of an illness. Patients also have the right to privacy and confidentiality (part of the medical profession's Hippocratic oath), the right to read their own medical records, and the right to receive emergency medical treatment regardless of ability to pay.

The legal rights of patients vary from state to state. Patients who are not satisfied with any aspect of their medical care, however, should always feel free to complain to their doctors or the hospital. In cases of serious neglect or misconduct, patients may also sue doctors or hospitals for *malpractice* or report them to state disciplinary boards for appropriate action.

▶ PEDIATRICIAN   see PHYSICIANS (M.D.'s)

▶ PHARMACIST

A pharmacist is a health-care professional who prepares and distributes medications prescribed by *physicians.* Pharmacists also play an important role in providing information, instructions, and advice about drugs to the general public. Most pharmacists work in pharmacies, or drugstores,

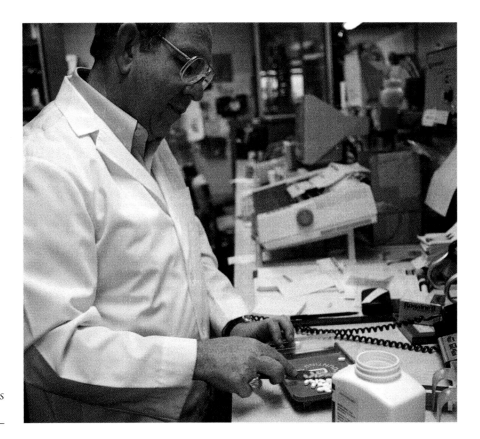

Filling a Prescription. *A pharmacist places the correct amount of medication in a container and labels it with detailed instructions on how to use the medication.*

but some work in hospitals, research laboratories, and the pharmaceutical industry.

The primary function of a pharmacist is to fill prescriptions written by physicians. For ready-made drugs, this involves measuring out the prescribed amount, putting it in a container, and writing a label that details how to take it. For certain prescriptions, the pharmacist must prepare the medication by compounding (mixing) the ingredients. Pharmacists may also keep computer records of all the medications taken by a client, called a *drug profile,* so that they can detect potential drug interactions or allergies. Pharmacists also advise customers about the purchase and use of nonprescription drugs, like cough syrups and cold medications, as well as the possibility of substituting a less-expensive generic drug for a name-brand medication.

People seeking a career as a pharmacist must complete a 5-year course at a college of pharmacy and a 1-year internship under the supervision of a practicing pharmacist. Pharmacists must also pass a state test to obtain a license to practice in the state. (See also PHYSICIANS (M.D.'s); DRUG INTERACTION, 7; GENERIC DRUGS, 7; NONPRESCRIPTION DRUGS, 7; PHARMACOLOGY, 7; PRESCRIPTION DRUGS, 7; SIDE EFFECTS, 7.)

▶ **PHYSICAL THERAPIST**   Physical therapists are professional HEALTH-CARE WORKERS who use a variety of techniques to help people cope with disabilities. They seek to reduce pain, restore mobility and strength, and teach people how to use devices such as wheelchairs, crutches, and walkers.

The techniques that physical therapists use include *active exercises*, in which the patients use stationary cycles, parallel bars, and pulleys and weights, and *passive exercises* in which the therapist moves the affected parts of the patient's body. Physical therapists also use cold packs to reduce swelling and heat treatments and massage to improve circulation and relieve pain. Whirlpool baths and electrical stimulation may also be used to relieve muscle pain.

Physical therapists usually work in a hospital or rehabilitation center. Their patients include people who have had surgery, who are recovering from injuries, or who have physically disabling diseases, such as muscular dystrophy, arthritis, or cerebral palsy. Typically, a physical therapist consults with a patient's physician, tests the patient, then designs a program tailored to meet the patient's needs.

People seeking to become physical therapists must complete college—either a 4-year college course in physical therapy or some other field of study plus an 18-month program to earn a physical therapy certificate. They must then pass a state licensing test to become certified to practice in their state. (See also HOME HEALTH SERVICES.)

▶ PHYSICIAN ASSISTANT

The physician assistant (P.A.) is a relatively new kind of health-care professional whose duties are somewhere between those of a doctor and those of a nurse. Physician assistants perform many of the routine medical tasks that doctors used to perform, allowing doctors to concentrate on more demanding aspects of medical practice. Working under the supervision of a doctor, a physician assistant takes medical histories, counsels patients, performs physical examinations, operates medical equipment, and takes specimens for laboratory tests.

People who want to become physician assistants must have at least 2 years of college. They must then complete a 2-year training program offered by a college, medical school, or hospital. Physician assistants are expected to be in great demand over the next decade. Many now work for the federal government or for large health-care providers like HEALTH MAINTENANCE ORGANIZATIONS (HMOs).

▶ PHYSICIANS (M.D.'s)

Physicians, or medical doctors, are individuals who are trained and licensed to practice medicine. Physicians diagnose and treat injuries and disease and promote good health practice. They are among the only health-care professionals who can prescribe medications and perform surgery.

In the United States, there are two types of medical degrees, the Doctor of Medicine (M.D.), conferred at most medical schools, and the Doctor of Osteopathy (D.O.), conferred at 15 osteopathic medical colleges. The training is basically equivalent, and both M.D.'s and D.O.'s can become licensed to practice in any area of medicine. More than 90

MEDICAL SPECIALTY BOARDS*

American Board of . . .

Allergy & Immunology	Otolaryngology
Anesthesiology	Pathology
Colon & Rectal Surgery	Pediatrics
Dermatology	Physical Medicine & Rehabilitation
Emergency Medicine	Plastic Surgery
Family Practice	Preventive Medicine
Internal Medicine	Psychiatry & Neurology
Neurological Surgery	Radiology
Nuclear Medicine	Surgery
Obstetrics & Gynecology	Thoracic (chest) Surgery
Ophthalmology	Urology
Orthopedic Surgery	

* The main specialty areas of medicine are governed by 23 boards, each composed of expert physicians in the particular field. Each board evaluates and certifies M.D.'s who want to practice in its area. Within these 23 board specialties are more than 80 practice specialties and subspecialties.

percent of physicians are M.D.'s. The following discussion generally refers to the training and specialties of M.D.'s. (See also OSTEOPATHIC PHYSICIANS (D.O.'s).

People planning to become physicians must complete 4 years of college and 4 years of medical school. The M.D. must then complete 1 year of postgraduate training (called an internship) in a hospital; this is usually followed by 2 to 6 more years of training (called a residency) in a specialty area. Before a physician can practice, he or she must pass a state examination to be licensed to practice in a particular state. Physicians may also take an examination to become certified by the national board in their specialty. Most physicians take continuing education courses to keep their licenses and to stay current with the latest medical findings and procedures.

Today, there are 23 main specialties, including the primary care areas (family practice, internal medicine, and pediatrics) as well as particular concentration on a major group of diseases or a specific body system (see chart: Medical Specialty Boards). Following are the areas of medicine covered by the major specialties.

Primary Care Physicians Primary care physicians provide regular medical checkups and broad-based medical care for most illnesses and injuries. When a primary care physician diagnoses a disease that requires surgery or specialized care, he or she generally refers the patient to a specialist.

▶ *Family Practitioners* (once called general practitioners, or G.P.'s) provide general care for people of all ages. A family practitioner may also be a specialist in internal medicine, pediatrics, or obstetrics/gynecology.

- *Internists* specialize in internal medicine—the diagnosis and non-surgical treatment of diseases in adults. Some internists treat routine illnesses in a general practice; others specialize in a particular area, such as the heart, digestive tract, or glands.
- *Pediatricians* specialize in the care of children from birth through adolescence. They measure the physical and emotional development of their patients and identify health problems. They also vaccinate children at specified ages to prevent diseases like measles and polio.

Specialists   Specialists provide what is referred to as secondary care. They are usually seen only when a patient has a condition that a primary care physician is not equipped to handle. Following are several of the major types of specialists.

> Specialists are usually seen only when a patient has a condition that a primary care physician is not equipped to handle.

- *Allergists* evaluate and treat sensitivities to substances, food, or environmental factors that cause allergic reactions.
- *Anesthesiologists* administer drugs to sedate or anesthetize patients during surgery and monitor the drugs' effects on the patient. (See also ANESTHESIOLOGIST.)
- *Cardiologists* diagnose and treat diseases and abnormalities of the heart and blood vessels. (See also HEART DISEASE, 3.)
- *Dermatologists* diagnose and treat diseases and disorders of the skin, hair, and nails.
- *Emergency Medicine Specialists* deal with the treatment of acute illnesses and injuries in emergency rooms or trauma centers.
- *Gastroenterologists* focus on treating diseases and disorders of the digestive system.
- *Geriatric Specialists* treat diseases and disorders of the elderly.
- *Hematologists* diagnose and treat disorders of the blood.
- *Immunologists* specialize in the functioning and disorders of the immune system.
- *Nephrologists* treat kidney diseases and disorders. (See also KIDNEY DISORDERS, 3.)
- *Neurologists* diagnose and treat diseases and injuries that affect the brain and nervous system.
- *Obstetrician/Gynecologists* specialize in treating women's reproductive systems. A gynecologist treats disorders of the reproductive organs; an obstetrician specializes in caring for pregnant women and delivering babies.
- *Oncologists* diagnose malignant growths and tumors and recommend cancer treatments, such as surgery, radiation therapy, and chemotherapy. (See also CANCER, 3.)
- *Ophthalmologists* treat poor vision with corrective glasses and diseases of the eye with medication or surgery. (See also EYE CARE.)
- *Orthopedists* treat injuries and structural disorders of the bones and joints.
- *Otolaryngologists* specialize in treating problems of the ear, nose, and throat.
- *Pathologists* study the causes and progress of diseases by examining specimens of body tissues, fluids, and secretions. (See also PATHOLOGIST.)

- *Psychiatrists* treat mental and emotional disorders through psychotherapy and by prescribing various medications. (See also PSYCHOTHERAPISTS.)
- *Radiologists* use technologies such as X-ray and ultrasound examinations to diagnose medical problems. Radiologists also use radiation to treat certain types of cancer. (See also RADIOLOGIST.)
- *Urologists* diagnose and treat disorders of the male and female urinary tract, as well as problems in the male reproductive system.

Choosing a Physician When choosing a primary care physician or a specialist, there are many factors to consider. Most important is a physician's abilities, which can be determined by checking his or her educational background, membership in professional associations, and board certification and by asking friends and other physicians for recommendations. It is also important to determine if the physician is easily accessible, has staff privileges at a convenient hospital, and has colleagues to care for patients when he or she is unavailable. Another consideration may be whether or not payment can be arranged conveniently through a patient's insurance.

A further important factor in choosing a physician is the rapport that develops between a physician and patient. A patient should feel comfortable confiding in the doctor and should find that the doctor listens carefully, responds thoughtfully, and gives instructions that are easy to understand. For help in choosing a doctor or determining the type of specialist needed, patients can turn to referral services offered by many hospitals and state and local medical societies. (See also GENETIC COUNSELOR; HEALTH-CARE SYSTEM; PREVENTIVE MEDICINE; SURGEON.)

▶ PODIATRIST

A podiatrist is a doctor who specializes in diagnosing, treating, and preventing disorders of the feet. Podiatrists treat ailments such as corns, bunions, calluses, and walking disorders in children. They also treat ankle and foot injuries in athletes and infections and ulcers of the feet. People who have diabetes are particularly prone to such infections. Podiatrists are trained to use a wide variety of methods to treat foot problems, including physical therapy, medication, corrective shoes, and surgery.

Most podiatrists complete college and a 4-year program at an accredited school of podiatry to become a doctor of podiatric medicine (D.P.M.). After graduating, podiatrists must pass an examination in order to be licensed to practice in their state. Some states also require a 1-year residency training program. A family doctor or local medical society can provide help in selecting a podiatrist. (See also FOOT PROBLEMS, **3.**)

▶ PREVENTIVE MEDICINE

Preventive medicine is a specialty area of medicine that focuses on the prevention or early detection of disease. Many *physicians* who specialize in preventive medicine are involved in *public health*, the promotion of the general health of a community. Government agencies

and other public health institutions work to prevent diseases in a community by such means as immunizing children against childhood diseases, supplying sanitation and a clean water supply, ensuring environmental safety, and providing health education.

Preventive medicine is also concerned with measures that the medical community or individuals can undertake to prevent disease. These include medical checkups, good prenatal care, and screening programs for diseases like cancer and heart disease. Also included is reducing the risk factors for disease through, for example, regular exercise, a good diet, and avoiding tobacco and the overuse of alcohol.

Some physicians in preventive medicine work with industry in the field of *occupational medicine.* They focus on preventing on-the-job accidents and diseases that result from workplace hazards like toxic chemicals. (See also DEPARTMENT OF HEALTH AND HUMAN SERVICES; OSTEOPATHIC PHYSICIANS (D.O.'s); PHYSICIANS (M.D.'s).)

▶ **PSYCHIATRIST**   see PSYCHOTHERAPISTS

▶ **PSYCHOLOGIST**   see PSYCHOTHERAPISTS

▶ **PSYCHOTHERAPISTS**   Psychotherapists are health-care professionals who help people with mental and emotional problems. They use *psychotherapy,* a method that involves talking about problems and symptoms with the patient, to change unhealthy ways of thinking and behaving. Health-care professionals who practice psychotherapy include psychiatrists, psychoanalysts, psychologists, social workers, and counselors.

Aims of Psychotherapy   In general, psychotherapists try to systematically lead patients to a better understanding of their problems through in-depth discussions. The goals are to improve counterproductive ways of thinking, feeling, and behaving that have developed over the years and to give patients more control over their lives. Psychotherapy can be provided individually, to couples or families, or to groups with similar problems. Specific approaches to therapy differ, depending on the type of psychotherapy practiced by the psychotherapist. There are four main types of psychotherapy: psychoanalytic, cognitive, behavioral, and humanistic. (See also PSYCHOTHERAPY, 5.)

Psychotherapists must provide an environment that encourages patients to express their emotions. The most successful psychotherapists share certain characteristics: They show warmth, caring, and empathy—

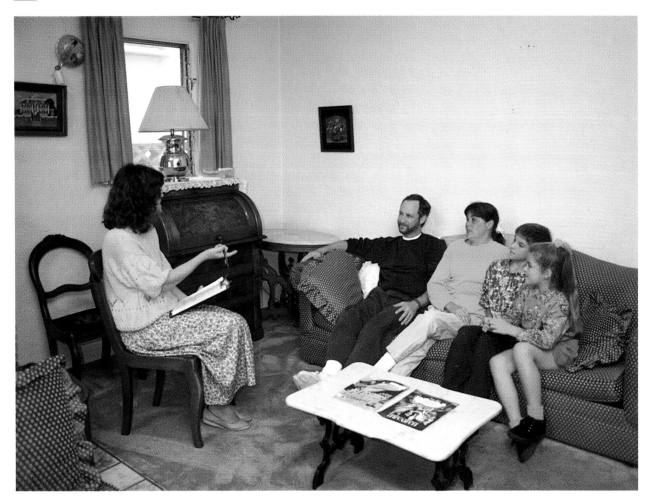

Psychotherapist. *Psychotherapists provide support and counseling to individuals, couples and families, and groups of people with similar problems.*

an understanding of the problems and feelings of others. Psychotherapists must also be reasonably free of emotional problems themselves, so that they can better concentrate on the problems of others.

Types of Psychotherapists *Psychiatrists* are *physicians* who have specialized in psychiatry by completing additional training in mental health. Because of their medical training, they are qualified to prescribe drugs as part of therapy. Most *psychoanalysts* are psychiatrists (and some are nonphysicians) who have completed training (usually at a psychoanalytic institute) in a theory of analysis that looks for the unconscious conflicts that are the root of emotional problems. This theory is based on the teachings of Dr. Sigmund Freud, a pioneer in the field of psychotherapy. *Psychologists* have earned a master's or doctoral degree from graduate schools of psychology. Because they do not have medical training, psychologists are not qualified to prescribe medication as a part of therapy. *Psychiatric social workers* have earned at least a master's degree from a graduate school of social work. Most work in hospitals, clinics, family service agencies, and schools. They may also work in private practice. *Counselors* usually have earned a master's or doctoral degree in counseling. They often work in schools or for religious organizations. Counselors refer people with serious problems to psychologists or psychiatrists. (See also PHYSICIANS (M.D.'s); PSYCHIATRY, **5**; PSYCHOLOGY, **5**.)

▷ **PUBLIC HEALTH SERVICE**   see DEPARTMENT OF HEALTH AND HUMAN SERVICES

▷ **QUACKERY**

Quackery involves selling worthless, even harmful, remedies or treatments for illness and injury. In most cases, quacks are completely unqualified individuals who claim to have medical skills. They promote worthless cures by taking advantage of the fear people have of being unattractive or of suffering pain, disability, or death. People with chronic, painful, or life-threatening diseases are the most vulnerable to quackery.

Quackery has been around for centuries. In the 1800s, "snake oil" salesmen used to travel from town to town hawking their so-called universal elixirs to unsuspecting victims. Although the government has done much to curb quacks, they still abound, and they have become much more sophisticated. Today, Americans spend as much as $25 billion a year on quack medicines, devices, and procedures.

Cancer Quackery   Cancer kills hundreds of thousands of Americans every year. Chemotherapy and radiation, the most successful treatments to combat cancer, are usually long and unpleasant. In recent years, quacks have enticed patients with cancer with quick, painless "miracle" remedies like laetrile, a poisonous substance derived from apricot pits, and megavitamin therapy. Not only are these remedies useless, they also may cause patients with cancer to delay getting effective treatment until the disease has progressed too far.

Quack Remedies. *Quack remedies have been around for years; and despite major efforts to educate the public and prevent quackery, Americans still spend billions of dollars each year on useless remedies.*

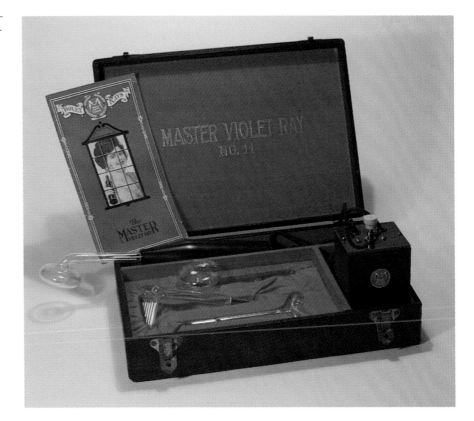

Arthritis Quackery   More than 20 million Americans have arthritis, a painful, chronic condition. Some worthless remedies, such as wearing a copper bracelet or having a bee sting the affected joint, are usually harmless. Other treatments can be dangerous. One so-called arthritis cure involves application of DMSO, an industrial solvent that is toxic in large amounts.

Weight-Loss Quackery   Obese or overweight people spend more than $100 million a year on bogus weight-reduction remedies. Quacks always promise that their pills, powders, or programs will make weight loss quick and easy. In some cases, the "miraculous weight-loss system" does work to some extent, because it includes the promotion of a low-fat, low-calorie diet that would have resulted in weight reduction without the quackery. (See also FAD DIETS, **4.**)

How to Spot Quackery   It is important to distinguish between quackery and unproved cures. An unproved cure may be a promising legitimate treatment for a disease that has not yet been subjected to adequate scientific testing. Most quack cures have been tested and have proved to be ineffective.

Beware of any medical cure that is advertised as guaranteed, secret, quick, or painless. Check the promoter's background with your local medical society or in medical directories usually found at the library. Look for information about the product in publications of the Food and Drug Administration (FDA) and the Federal Trade Commission (FTC). Many quacks falsely claim to be physicians or have phony degrees. Avoid products and procedures that are advertised in supermarket tabloids. Usually, these ads include dramatic "before" and "after" photos of someone who allegedly has been helped by the product.

One common tactic used by promoters of quack remedies is to claim that they are victims of a conspiracy by the medical establishment. The quack usually claims that orthodox doctors fear losing income and patients once the public becomes aware of the new miracle cure. Another common sign of quackery is that the quack operates a clinic or office outside the jurisdiction of federal and state governments. Most laetrile clinics, for example, were located just across the Mexican border from the United States.

Quack remedies sometimes seem to work because the patient may coincidentally experience a remission of the disease while trying the product or service. The patient may believe that the "miracle" remedy was the cause. Sometimes quack treatments have a placebo effect. This means that they seem to work because the person receiving them believes they do. (See also PLACEBO, **7.**)

> Beware of any medical cure that is advertised as guaranteed, secret, quick, or painless. Check the promoter's background with your local medical society.

▶ **RADIOLOGIST**   Radiologists are physicians who specialize in using imaging techniques to diagnose and treat disease. The imaging techniques include X rays, ultrasound, CAT scans, magnetic resonance imaging, and radioactive substances. By using these techniques, physicians can locate and identify

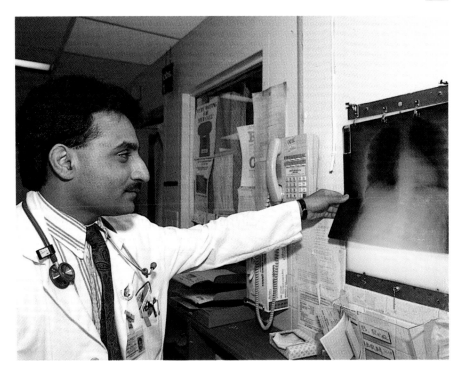

Evaluating an X ray. *Radiologists use various imaging techniques to diagnose and treat diseases and disorders.*

disorders, often eliminating the need for exploratory surgery or other invasive procedures. Radiologists also use radiation to treat cancer.

Some radiologists work in hospitals whereas others run private radiology centers. Radiologists must complete 4 years of medical school and at least 5 years of training in their medical specialty. (See also PHYSICIANS (M.D.'s); MAGNETIC RESONANCE IMAGING, 3; RADIATION THERAPY, 3; X-RAY EXAMINATION, 3; ULTRASOUND, 6; RADIATION, 8.)

▶ REGISTERED NURSE   see NURSING

▶ REHABILITATION CENTER

A rehabilitation center is a health-care facility designed to help people recover the physical abilities they have lost through injury or illness. For example, an athlete with a torn tendon might receive physical therapy, whereas a person who has had a stroke might receive both physical and speech therapy. Some centers also offer occupational therapy, which helps people relearn daily tasks. Hearing therapy and psychotherapy might also be offered.

Some rehabilitation centers are part of a hospital, used both by hospital patients and by outpatients. Skilled-care nursing homes sometimes contain rehabilitation centers focused primarily on therapy for the elderly. Independent rehabilitation centers may deal with various types of disability or specialize in one type. For example, sports medicine centers treat people with sports-related injuries.

A different type of rehabilitation center focuses on helping people recover from a dependency on alcohol or drugs. These centers provide counseling and support during withdrawal and recovery. (See also NURSING HOME; OCCUPATIONAL THERAPIST; PHYSICAL THERAPIST; SPEECH THERAPY; PSYCHOTHERAPY, 5; DRUG REHABILITATION, 7.)

▶ SOCIAL WORKER   see PSYCHOTHERAPISTS

▶ SPEECH THERAPY

Speech therapy is the treatment of speech and language disorders, such as stuttering, lisping, slurred speech, and problems with voice production. These disorders may be caused by birth defect, injury, illness, emotional problems, or hearing loss. Experts in speech therapy, called *speech-language pathologists*, use a variety of specialized techniques to help improve speech and communication.

The speech-language pathologist usually begins therapy by performing diagnostic tests and taking a case history to learn as much as possible

Speech Therapy. *Therapy for speech and language disorders may include a program of exercises to correct the problem. The therapist may also involve the family and others in the treatment process.*

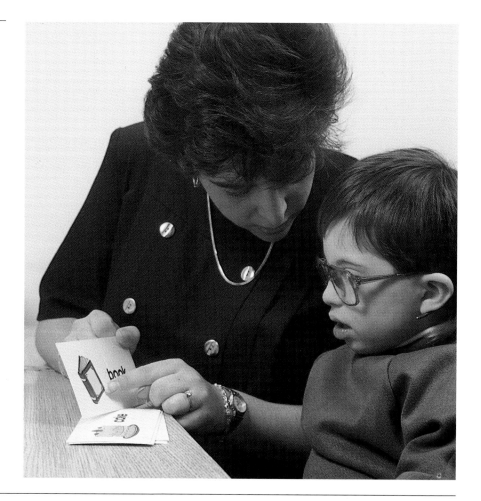

about how and when the problem began. The speech-language pathologist may consult with the individual's physician or psychologist to help assess and diagnose the problem. The speech-language pathologist then decides on a form of treatment that takes into account the case history and type of disorder, as well as such factors as the individual's age and special needs. Therapy usually includes a program of exercises to correct defective speech and learn new speech or language skills. The therapist also tries to involve people who have close contact, such as family, teachers, and friends, in the treatment process.

To become a speech-language pathologist, a person usually must have a master's degree in speech-language pathology. Many speech-language pathologists work for public school systems; others work for hospitals, universities, or government agencies or have private practices. (See also SPEECH DISORDERS, 3.)

▶ SURGEON

Surgeons are *physicians* who perform procedures that involve opening up the body (*surgery*) to treat disease and repair injuries and deformities. They first examine the patient to determine whether surgery is necessary by evaluating the patient's medical history and general health. Surgeons also estimate the risks of surgery and determine the best surgical approach.

A *general surgeon* performs many types of operations. *Specialists* in surgery concentrate on a particular branch of surgery. For example, an orthopedic surgeon treats injuries and diseases of the bones and joints, a neurosurgeon operates on the brain and spinal cord, and a plastic surgeon corrects superficial problems of the face and body.

To become a surgeon, 4 years of medical school and at least 5 years of additional training in surgery are required. (See also DENTAL CARE—ORAL SURGEON; PHYSICIANS (M.D.'s); SURGERY, 3.)

▶ THERAPIST

see PSYCHOTHERAPISTS

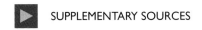

SUPPLEMENTARY SOURCES

Aaseng, Nathan. 1987. *The disease fighters: The Nobel Prize in medicine.* Minneapolis, Minn.: Lerner Publications Co.

Altman, Nathaniel. 1990. *Everybody's guide to chiropractic health care.* Los Angeles: Jeremy P. Tarcher.

Bleich, Alan R. 1988. *Exploring careers in medicine.* New York: Rosen Publishing Group.

Career information center, 5th ed. Volume 7: Health. 1993. New York: Macmillan.

Colen, B. D. 1986. *Hard choices: Mixed blessings of modern medical technology.* New York: Putnam.

Dixon, Bernard, ed. 1986. *Health, medicine, and the human body.* New York: Macmillan.

Franck, Irene M., and David M. Brownstone. 1989. *Healers.* New York: Facts On File.

Heron, Jackie. 1987. *Exploring careers in nursing.* New York: Rosen Publishing Group.

McGrew, Roderick E. 1985. *Encyclopedia of medical history.* New York: McGraw-Hill.

Olsen, Kristin G. 1989. *The encyclopedia of alternative health care.* New York: Pocket Books.

Reese, Alan M., and Catherine Hoffman. 1990. *Consumer health information sourcebook,* 3d ed. Phoenix, Ariz.: Oryx Press.

Stanfield, Peggy. 1990. *Introduction to the health professions.* Boston: Jones & Bartlett.

ORGANIZATIONS

American Academy of Ophthalmology
655 Beach Street
San Francisco, CA 94109
(415) 561-8500

American Academy of Pediatrics
141 Northwest Point Boulevard
P.O. Box 927
Elk Grove Village, IL 60009
(708) 228-5005

American Chiropractic Association
1701 Clarendon Boulevard
Arlington, VA 22209
(202) 276-8800

American Dental Association
211 East Chicago Avenue
Chicago, IL 60611
(312) 440-2500

American Health Care Association
1201 L Street, NW
Washington, DC 20005
(202) 842-4444

American Holistic Medical Association
4101 Lake Boone Trail
Suite 201
Raleigh, NC 27607
(919) 787-5146

American Hospital Association
840 North Lake Shore Drive
Chicago, IL 60611
(312) 280-6000

American Medical Association
515 North State Street
Chicago, IL 60610
(312) 464-5000

American Nurses' Association
2420 Pershing Road
Kansas City, MO 64108
(816) 474-5720

American Osteopathic Association
142 East Ontario Street
Chicago, IL 60611
(312) 280-5800

American Physical Therapy Association
1111 North Fairfax Street
Alexandria, VA 22314
(703) 684-2782

American Psychiatric Association
1400 K Street, NW
Washington, DC 20005
(202) 682-6000

American Psychological Association
1200 Seventeenth Street, NW
Washington, DC 20036
(202) 336-5500

Hospice Association of America
519 C Street, NE
Washington, DC 20002
(202) 546-4759

National Emergency Medicine Association
306 West Joppa Road
Towson, MD 21204
(301) 494-0300

INDEX

Italicized page numbers refer to illustrations or charts.

AA. *See* Alcoholics Anonymous (AA)
Abdomen, **1**:4. *See also* Gallbladder,
  1:42–43; Kidney, **1**:57–58; Liver,
  1:60–62; Pancreas, **1**:76–77
Abdominal hysterectomy, **6**:48, *48*
Abortion, **6**:4–5, *75*
  medical ethics dealing with, **9**:21
  See also Contraception, **6**:24–26;
    Female reproductive system,
    6:33–34; Fetus, **6**:37–38; Ge-
    netic screening, **6**:42–44; Mis-
    carriage, **6**:61–62
Abrasions, **4**:103–4, **8**:101
Abscess, **2**:4, *4*, 51
  in tooth, **3**:44–45, *45*
  See also Boil, **2**:15–16; Infection,
    2:50–51; Pus, **2**:74–75
Absences (petit mal seizures), **3**:54
Abstinence, **6**:5
  from alcohol, **7**:14
  from sexual intercourse, **6**:5, 24,
    83, 95
  See also Menstruation, **6**:59–61;
    Natural family planning, **6**:66;
    Safer sex, **6**:82–83; Sexual in-
    tercourse, **6**:91–92
Abuse. *See* Drug use and abuse,
  7:55–57; Child abuse, **8**:22–23;
  Spouse abuse, **8**:86
Acceptance of death, **5**:40–41
Access for people with disabilities,
  8:4–5
Accidental amputation, **3**:10
Accidents, **8**:5–6
  alcohol-related, **7**:46–47
  of children, **8**:5, 6, 14, 53
  death by, **8**:5, *6*, 12, 14, 26, 51,
    98
  with electricity, **8**:30–31, 52
  firearm, **8**:46
  in home, **8**:5, 6, 51–53, *52*, 67,
    68, 69
  on the job, **8**:5, 59, 79, 80
  noise level and, **8**:59
  nuclear, **8**:62
  preventing, **8**:6
  reasons for, **8**:5–6
  types of, **8**:5, *6*
  See also Automobile safety,
    8:11–13; Bicycle safety, **8**:14;
    Drowning, **8**:26–27; Motor-

cycle safety, **8**:58; Water safety,
  8:98–99
Accutane, **7**:19
ACE (angiotensin-converting en-
  zyme) inhibitors, **7**:27
Acetaminophen, **7**:16
Achilles tendon, **1**:10, 41
Acid indigestion, **7**:18
Acid rain, **8**:6–7, *7*
  air pollution and, **8**:6–7, 9–10
  fossil fuels and, **8**:6–7, *7*, 40
  water pollution from, **8**:95
  See also Particulates, **8**:65–66
Acne, **1**:90, **3**:4–5, *4*
  antiacne agents to treat, **7**:19
  See also Skin, **1**:89–90; Puberty,
    6:79–80
Acquaintance rape. *See* Date rape
Acquired immunity, **2**:47
Acquired immunodeficiency syn-
  drome. *See* AIDS
ACTH (adrenocorticotropic hor-
  mone), **1**:80, *80*, **3**:90
Active exercises, **9**:31
Active immunity, **2**:47, 48
Active prevention of accidents, **8**:6
Active protection in safety equip-
  ment, **8**:77
Active solar energy systems, **8**:84
Acupuncture, **1**:37, **3**:5–6, **9**:4, *4*
  endorphins released during, **3**:5,
    7:87
  quitting smoking and, **7**:87
Acute bronchitis, **2**:17
Acute diarrhea, **2**:30
Acute glaucoma, **3**:60
Acute lymphoblastic leukemia (ALL),
  3:84
Acute myeloblastic leukemia (AML),
  3:84
Acute sinusitis, **2**:84
Acyclovir, **2**:6, 44, 45, 84, **7**:29
Adam's apple, **1**:96
Addict/codependent relationship,
  7:39–40
Addiction, **7**:4–5, 85
  Alcoholics Anonymous and
    breaking, **7**:9–12
  alcoholism, **7**:12–14
  to cigarettes, **7**:85–87
  to cocaine, **7**:37–38

consequences of, **7**:5
drug rehabilitation programs for,
  7:5, 16, 49–50, 63, 74
illegal drug use and, **7**:54
signs of, **7**:5
stages of, **7**:4–5, 56–57
tolerance leading to, **7**:99
withdrawal syndrome and, **7**:4–5,
  57
See also Drug use and abuse,
  7:55–57; Psychoactive drugs,
  7:84–85; Smoking, **7**:90–92
Addison's disease, **1**:7
Additive effect of drugs, **7**:48
Additives, food, **4**:52–53
Adenoidectomy, **1**:5
Adenoids, **1**:4–5, *5. See also* Lymphatic system, **1**:63–64; Respiratory
  system, **1**:84–86; Sinus(es), **1**:88–89
Adhesions, **1**:87
Adjustment, **5**:4. *See also* Coping skills,
  5:29–30; Self-efficacy, **5**:88; Stress-
  management techniques, **5**:98–99
Adjuvant therapy
  for cancer, **3**:27, 31
  after mastectomy, **6**:57
Administrative dietitians, **9**:26
Adolescence, **1**:5–6, 78
  alienation in, **5**:6
  experimentation in, **5**:5
  friendship during, **5**:47
  gender identity in, **6**:40
  growth spurt in, **6**:84
  nocturnal emission in, **6**:54, 67, 80
  peer pressure in, **5**:67–68
  puberty and, **6**:79–80
  self-image and, **5**:90
  shifts in self-esteem in, **5**:89
  suicide during, **5**:99–100
  value development in, **5**:101
  See also Self-image, **5**:89–90; Fe-
    male reproductive system,
    6:33–34; Male reproductive
    system, **6**:52–54
Adoption, **6**:6–7. *See also* Teenage
  pregnancy, **6**:97–98
Adrenal cortex, **1**:6, 7, *7*
Adrenal glands, **1**:6–7, *7*
  and endocrine system, **1**:36
  hormones produced by, **1**:6, 7, *51*
  and kidney, **1**:57

See also Epinephrine, **1**:38–39; Nervous system, **1**:71–74; Stress, **5**:95–98

Adrenalin, **1**:39

Adrenaline. *See* Epinephrine

Adrenal medulla, **1**:6, 7, *7*

Adrenocorticotropic hormone (ACTH), **1**:80, *80,* **3**:90

Adulthood, **1**:8
stages of, **5**:5
See also Lifestyle, **4**:71–72; Heredity and environment, **5**:49–50

Adult identity, **5**:4–5. *See also* Developmental psychology, **5**:34–36; Responsibility, **5**:84–85; Self-actualization, **5**:87; Self-esteem, **5**:88–89; Values, **5**:100–101

Aerobic dance, **4**:4. *See also* Aerobic exercise, **4**:4–6; Endurance, **4**:34–35; Fitness training, **4**:49–50; Flexibility, **4**:51–52; Heart rate, **4**:68

Aerobic exercise, **4**:4–6, 39–40
cycling, **4**:25–26
endorphins and, **1**:37
endurance and, **4**:35, 50
fitness and, **4**:49
fitness training and, **4**:50
running, **4**:95–96
stress management with, **5**:98
swimming, **4**:112–13
training for sports and, **4**:100
walking, **4**:122–23
for weight management, **4**:132
See also Flexibility, **4**:51–52; Sports and fitness, **4**:99–101; Strength, **4**:107

Aerosols used as inhalants, **7**:66

Affective disorders, **5**:33–34

Afterbirth, **6**:72

Age
basal metabolic rate and, **4**:16
measurements of, **9**:13

Ageism, **5**:73

Agent-host-environment model, **7**:57

Age-related hearing loss, **3**:67

Agglutination, **1**:17

Aggressiveness, **5**:5–6, 7, 12–13. *See also* Alcoholism, **7**:12–14; Violence, **8**:92–93

Aging, **1**:8, 9
cataract formation and, **3**:35
gerontologists and study of, **9**:13
life expectancy and, **1**:59–60
menopause and, **6**:58–59
senility and, **5**:90–91

See also Diabetes, **3**:46–48; Genetics, **6**:40–42

Agricultural chemicals, **4**:6–7, 86, **8**:7. *See also* Food additives, **4**:52–53; Food safety, **4**:61–63

Agricultural pollution, **8**:7–8
of water, **8**:8, 95, 96
See also Agricultural chemicals, **4**:6–7; Organic food, **4**:86; Toxic substances, **8**:91–92

Agriculture, genetic engineering uses in, **8**:44

AIDS, **1**:14, 54, **2**:4–8, **3**:25, 75, 81–82, **6**:*94*
anal sex and transmission of, **6**:8
AZT to fight, **7**:29, 30, 31
diagnosing, **2**:6
HIV and, **2**:5, 45–46
Kaposi's sarcoma, **2**:46, **3**:81–82
prevention of, **2**:7–8, **6**:22–23
reported cases of (1982–1990), **2**:82
risk factors for, **2**:4–5, 7–8
safer sex and, **2**:7–8, 46, **6**:82–83
social consequences of, **2**:8
symptoms and course of, **2**:5–6, 7
transmission of, **2**:5, **7**:54, 56, 67, 77
treatment of, **2**:6–7
virus, **2**:5
See also Immune system, **1**:52–55; Pneumonia, **2**:72–73; Sexually transmitted diseases (STDs), **2**:82; Blood transfusion, **3**:25; STDs, **6**:94–95

AIDS dementia, **2**:6, **5**:66

AIDS-related complex (ARC), **2**:6

Air bags, **8**:12, 78

Airborne allergens, **3**:6

Air pollution, **8**:9–10, *10*
acid rain and, **8**:6–7, 9–10
carbon monoxide and, **8**:21
dealing with, **8**:10
ecosystem upset by, **8**:29
fossil fuels and, **8**:9, 40–41
health hazards caused by, **1**:85–86, **8**:100
particulates and, **8**:9, 66
reducing, **8**:33–34
smog and, **8**:9, 82
temperature inversion and, **8**:9, 90
toxic substances in, **8**:91
See also Asthma, **3**:17–19; Heart disease, **3**:69–72; Lung disease, **3**:85–87; Carbon dioxide, **8**:21; Ozone, **8**:64–65; Radon, **8**:74

Airway, checking and opening victim's, **8**:24, *25*

Al-Anon, **7**:11, 40

Alarm stage of general adaptation syndrome, **5**:96, 97

Alateen, **7**:11–12, 40

Alcohol, **7**:6–9
blood alcohol level (BAL), **7**:6, 7, 9, 33–34, 46, 68
cirrhosis and, **3**:38–39
dependence on, **7**:8, 14
drinking and driving, **7**:7, 8, 9, 46–47
drug interactions with, **7**:23, 26, 48
effects of, **7**:6–8, 9, *33,* 34
fetal alcohol syndrome and, **6**:12, 38, 78, **7**:58–59
hangover from, **7**:7, 61–62
intoxication from, **7**:7–8, 68–69
regulation of, **7**:53
social drinking of, **7**:12, 92–93
water safety and avoidance of, **8**:98
See also Antihistamines and decongestants, **7**:25–27; Drugs, **7**:50–52; Sedatives, **7**:87–88

Alcoholics Anonymous (AA), **7**:9–12, 14
Al-Anon and, **7**:11, 40
Alateen and, **7**:11–12, 40
getting help from, **7**:10–11
twelve steps of, **7**:9–10, *10*
See also Addiction, **7**:4–5; Alcoholism, **7**:12–14

Alcoholism, **1**:61–62, **7**:7–8, 12–14
aggressiveness and, **5**:6
causes of, **7**:12
cirrhosis and, **3**:38, 39
codependency and, **7**:39–40
delirium tremens and, **7**:42
malnutrition and, **4**:75
recognizing, **7**:14
social drinking and, **7**:12, 92–93
steps toward, **7**:12–14
treatment of, **7**:14, 18
violence and, **8**:92
See also Drug rehabilitation, **7**:49–50

Aldosterone, **1**:7, 51, *51*

Alienation, **5**:6

Alimentary canal, **1**:10, 30, 31, *31*

Alleles, **6**:40–41

Allergens, **3**:6, 8–9, 64, 79, **7**:25

Allergic rhinitis. *See* Hay fever

Allergies, **1**:54, 90, **3**:6–8
to antibiotics, **2**:9, **7**:21, 22
antihistamines and decongestants for, **7**:25–27

to antiserums, 2:11–12
bronchodilators to treat, 7:34
drug, 3:6, 7:47
food, 4:53–54
hay fever, 3:64–65
to insect repellents, 7:68
rashes and, 2:76
See also Immune system,
1:52–55; Conjunctivitis,
2:26–27; Asthma, 3:17–19;
Eczema, 3:51; Guillain-Barré
syndrome, 3:61–62
Allergists, 9:33
Allergy immunotherapy, 3:7, 79
Allergy tests, 3:8–9, 19
Alopecia. *See* Hair loss
Alpha-fetoprotein test, 6:44
Altered states of consciousness, 5:63
Alternative health care, 9:4, *4*
acupuncture, 3:5–6
chiropractic, 9:4, 5–6
Altruism. *See* Prosocial behavior
Alveoli, 1:63, 84, 3:53, *53*
Alzheimer's disease, 1:9, 74, 3:9–10,
43, 44
organic brain disorders and, 5:66
See also Brain, 1:19–21; Senility,
5:90–91
Amantadine, 7:29
Ambulance services, emergency, 8:32
Amebic dysentery, 2:31, 69
Amenorrhea, 6:60
American Association of Blood
Banks, 1:14
American Cancer Society, 3:30, 40
American Dental Association seal,
7:76
American Dietetic Association
(ADA), 9:26
American Heart Association, 8:25
American Medical Association, 7:46
American Psychiatric Association,
5:60
American Red Cross, 1:14, 8:25
Americans with Disabilities Act
(1990), 8:4
Amino acids, 4:14, 76, 90
Aminoglycosides, 7:21
Amnesia, 5:6–7
Amniocentesis, 3:50, 6:43, *43*, 78
ultrasound during, 6:43, 100
Amniotic fluid, 6:7, *7*, 20
amniocentesis and sample of,
6:43, *43*
See also Female reproductive sys-
tem, 6:33–34; Genetic screen-
ing, 6:42–44; Placenta,
6:71–72; Umbilical cord, 6:101
Amniotic sac, 6:7, 30, 74

Amoebas, abscess caused by, 2:4
Amoxicillin, 7:80
Amphetamines, 4:27, 7:15, 96
as appetite suppressant, 7:15
designer, 7:43
look-alike drugs mimicking, 7:70
See also Addiction, 7:4–5; Drugs
and the law, 7:53–54; Drug use
and abuse, 7:55–57; Ritalin,
7:87; Side effects, 7:89
Ampicillin, 7:80
Amputation, 3:10–11, 59
Amyl nitrate, 7:66
Anabolic steroids, 4:13, 7:94–95
Anabolism, 1:64, 4:15
Anaerobic bacteria, 2:89–90
Anaerobic exercise, 4:5, 7, 40. *See
also* Aerobic exercise, 4:4–6; Endurance, 4:34–35; Fitness,
4:48–49; Fitness training, 4:49–50;
Strength exercise, 4:108–9; Weight
training, 4:132–33
Analgesics, 3:94, 7:15–17, 51–52
as anti-inflammatory drugs, 7:28
aspirin, 7:30
comparing, 7:16
functioning of, 7:15–16
for influenza, 2:53
narcotic, 7:15–16, *16*
nonnarcotic, 7:15, *16*, 17
for sprains and strains, 8:87
supply in medicine cabinet, 7:73
See also Pain, 3:94; Addiction,
7:4–5; Cough medicine, 7:41;
Methadone, 7:74–75; Tolerance, 7:99
Anal sex, 2:7–8, 46, 6:8, 94. *See also*
AIDS, 2:4–8; Safer sex, 6:82–83
Anaphylactic shock, 3:6, 79, 101,
7:21, 25, 47
food allergy and, 4:53
insect bites and stings and, 8:17
Androgens, 1:7, 6:47, 84
acne and, 3:4
See also Sex hormones, 6:84–85
Anemia, 1:14, 16, 18, 69, 3:11–12,
102, 113, 115, 4:70, 117
aplastic, 1:18, 3:12
hookworm infestation and, 2:69
iron-deficiency, 3:11–12, 4:70
sickle cell, 3:102
See also Blood test, 1:16; Bone
marrow, 1:18–19; Iron,
4:69–70; Vitamin B complex,
4:116–17
Anesthesia, 3:12–13, *13*, 109. *See also*
Pain, 3:94; Anesthesiologist, 9:4–5
Anesthesiologist, 3:13, *13*, 9:4–5,
33. *See also* Anesthesia, 3:12–13;

Anesthetic drugs, 7:17; Nursing,
9:24–25
Anesthetic drug(s), 7:17, 9:20
alcohol as, 7:6
local anesthetic, 3:12–13, 7:17,
67, 9:4
See also Acupuncture, 3:5–6;
Anesthesia, 3:12–13; Anal-
gesics, 7:15–17; Anesthesiolo-
gist, 9:4–5
Anesthetists, 9:4–5, 24
Aneurysm, 1:12, 3:13–14, *14*, 107.
See also Arteriosclerosis, 3:15;
Blood clot, 3:24; Cardiovascular
disease, 3:34; Heart disease,
3:69–72; Hypertension, 3:77–78
Angel dust (PCP), 7:61
Anger, 5:7–8. *See also* Aggressiveness,
5:5–6; Assertiveness, 5:12–13; Con-
flict resolution, 5:27–28; Coping
skills, 5:29–30; Emotion, 5:42–44;
Personality(ies), 5:69–70
Anger stage of dying, 5:40
Angina pectoris, 3:69, 7:32
Angiography, 3:14, 19
Angioplasty, 3:19, 69, 74
Angiotensin-converting enzyme
(ACE) inhibitors, 7:27
Animal bites, 8:15–16, 17, 55
Animal research, 9:22
Ankle, 1:9–10, *10*
sprained, 8:87
See also Connective tissue,
1:27–28; Joint(s), 1:56;
Musculoskeletal system,
1:68–69
Annatto extract, 4:53
Anopheles mosquito, 2:59
Anorexia, 4:8, 33–34, *33*, 5:8
Anorgasmia, 6:89
Antabuse, 7:18, 50. *See also* Drug re-
habilitation, 7:49–50; Withdrawal
syndrome, 7:100–101
Antacids, 3:106, 7:18–19
drug interaction with, 7:48
supply in medicine cabinet, 7:73
See also Stomachache/indiges-
tion, 3:105–6; Ulcer, peptic,
3:114–15
Antagonism, drug, 7:48
Anterior lobe (pituitary), 1:80
Antiacne agents, 7:19. *See also* Acne,
3:4–5
Antianxiety drugs, 5:39, *39*, 40, 81
Antibiotic ointment, 7:20, 73. *See
also* Bacterial infections, 2:13–15
Antibiotics, 7:20–22, 52
drug interactions with, 7:23, 48
penicillin, 7:80

problems associated with, 7:21
resistance to, 7:21–22
types of, 7:21
See also Antibiotic treatment,
2:8–10; Bacterial infections,
2:13–15; Candida infections,
2:19; Antifungal agents,
7:24–25; Antiviral drugs,
7:29–30
Antibiotic treatment, 2:8–10
for bacterial infections, 2:14, 64
for chlamydial infections, 2:21
functioning of, 2:9
with penicillin, 7:80
problems and resistance to,
2:9–10
for streptococcal infections, 2:86,
87
for syphilis, 2:88
for tuberculosis, 2:95
See also Culture, 2:28–29; Antibiotics, 7:20–22
Antibody(ies), 1:53–54, 2:10,
3:61–62, 64, 80
antigen-antibody reaction, 2:10,
11
autoimmune disorders and, 2:51
in breast milk, 4:18, 19
food allergies and, 4:53
in gamma globulin, 2:39
HIV antibody testing, 2:6, 46
immunity and, 2:47
for newborn baby, 6:38
viral infection and, 2:97, 98
See also Immune system,
1:52–55; Immunization,
2:47–49
Anticancer drugs, 7:22–23
chemotherapy, 3:37
interferon, 2:53–54
See also Cancer, 3:29–32; Radiation therapy, 3:99; Hormone
therapy, 7:63–64
Anticoagulants, 3:24, 107, 7:23. *See
also* Blood clot, 3:24; Heart attack,
3:68–69; Stroke, 3:106–8; Drug
interaction, 7:47–48
Antidepressants, 5:39, *39,* 81,
7:23–24. *See also* Depression,
5:32–34; Drug interaction,
7:47–48; Psychoactive drugs,
7:84–85
Antidiarrheal products, 7:24, 73. *See
also* Diarrhea, 2:29–30
Antidiuretic hormone (ADH), 1:80,
80
Antidotes, 7:49
Antifungal agents, 7:24–25. *See also*
Fungal infections, 2:38–39

Antigen, 1:17, 53–54, 2:10–11. *See
also* Immune system, 1:52–55;
Antibody(ies), 2:10; Microorganisms, 2:63–65; Toxin, 2:94
Antigen-antibody reaction, 2:10, *11*
Antihistamines and decongestants,
3:7, 65, 7:25–27, *26*
for allergies, 7:25–27
antihistamine as sleep remedy,
7:90
caffeine in, 7:35
for common colds, 2:24
drug interactions with, 7:26, 48
eyedrops, 7:58
for motion sickness, 8:58
supply in medicine cabinet, 7:73
See also Hay fever, 3:64–65
Antihormones, 7:22
Antihypertensives, 3:78, 7:27
diuretics as, 7:27, 44
See also Heart disease, 3:69–72;
Hypertension, 3:77–78
Anti-inflammatory drugs, 7:28, 30
aspirin as, 7:28, 30
See also Inflammation, 2:51–52;
Corticosteroids, 7:40; Non-
prescription drugs, 7:78–79;
Prescription drugs, 7:82–83
Antimicrobials, 4:52
Antioxidants, 4:10, 52, 89, 117, 119
Antiperspirants, 7:42
Antipsychotic drugs, 5:39, *39,* 40, 81,
86
Antirabies vaccine, 2:75
Antisepsis, 8:81, 9:20
Antiseptics, 2:15, 3:109, 7:28–29, 73,
8:81. *See also* Infection, 2:50–51
Antiserum, 2:11–12. *See also* Gamma
globulin, 2:39; Immunization,
2:47–49; Microorganisms, 2:63–65
Antismoking products, 7:87
Antisocial personality, 5:9, 71. *See
also* Aggressiveness, 5:5–6
Antitoxins, 2:11, 31, 94
Antiviral drugs, 7:29–30. *See also*
AIDS, 2:4–8; Viral infections,
2:97–98
Anus, 1:10–11
hemorrhoids in lining of, 3:75
itching around, 2:54
pinworms in, 2:69
See also Rectum, 1:81
Anvil (incus), 1:33, 34
Anxiety, 5:9–10
desensitization to overcome,
5:17–18
sexual dysfunction and, 6:89
See also Anxiety disorders,
5:10–12; Drug therapy,

5:39–40; Sleep problems,
5:93–94
Anxiety disorders, 5:10–12, 39. *See
also* Behavior modification, 5:16–18;
Coping skills, 5:29–30; Drug ther-
apy, 5:39–40; Psychotherapy,
5:79–82; Relaxation training, 5:84
Anxiolytics (antianxiety drugs), 7:87,
90
Aorta, 1:11, *11,* 12, 26, *26,* 48
aneurysm in, 3:13, 14
See also Artery(ies), 1:12; Circu-
latory system, 1:25–27; Ather-
osclerosis, 3:19–20;
Hypertension, 3:77–78
Apgar, Virginia, 6:8
Apgar test, 6:8–9, *8. See also* Child-
birth, 6:20–21
Aphasia, 3:104
Aplastic anemia, 1:18, 3:12
Apnea, sleep, 1:92, 3:103, 104
Appendectomy, 3:14
Appendicitis, 1:11, 3:14
Appendix, 1:11, *11,* 3:14, *14*
Appetite, 4:8, 68
hunger versus, 4:68–69
See also Thyroid disorders, 3:112;
Diets, 4:30–32; Eating dis-
orders, 4:33–34; Food craving,
4:54–55; Weight management,
4:130–32; Anorexia/bulimia,
5:8
Appetite suppressant(s), 4:8, 27,
7:43–44, 95
amphetamines as, 7:15
nicotine as, 7:98
Aqueous humor, 3:60
Aquifers, 8:94
ARC (AIDS-related complex), 2:6
Arches of foot, 1:42, 3:57
Areola, 6:13
Arm (subaxillary) temperature, 8:19
Arousal, sexual, 6:33, 93
Arrhythmia, 3:68, 71
Arterial bleeding, 8:18
Arteriosclerosis, 1:9, 3:13, 15, 69. *See
also* Artery, 1:12; Atherosclerosis,
3:19–20; Gangrene, 3:59; Heart
attack, 3:68–69; Hypertension,
3:77–78; Stroke, 3:106–8; Cholesterol, 4:23–24
Artery(ies), 1:12, *12, 26,* 3:19
aorta, 1:11
diseases of, 3:13–14, 15, 19–20,
34
hepatic, 1:61
pulmonary, 1:12, *26,* 48
radial, taking pulse in, 8:72
umbilical, 6:101

See also Circulatory system, 1:25–27; Atherosclerosis, 3:19–20; Hypertension, 3:77–78

Arthritis, 1:9, 46, 69, 3:15–17, 22, 58, 98
  anti-inflammatory drugs for, 7:28
  gout, 1:42
  Lyme disease and, 2:58–59
  rheumatoid, 1:28, 50, 56, 59, 69, 88, 3:16–17
  temporomandibular joint (TMJ) syndrome, 1:55, 3:110–11
  See also Aging, 1:9; Connective tissue, 1:27–28; Joint, 1:56

Arthritis quackery, 9:38
Arthroscopy, 3:109
Articulation disorder, 3:104
Artificial heart implantation, 3:74
Artificial insemination, 6:51
Artificial limb, 3:10, 10
Artificial pacemaker implantation, 3:74
Artificial respiration, 8:22. *See also* CPR, 8:24–25
Artificial sweeteners, 4:8–9, 11, 52. *See also* Diet food, 4:29–30; Sugar, 4:110–11
Artificial tears, 7:58
Asbestos, 8:10–11
  removal of, 3:33, 33
  See also Carcinogens, 3:33; Lung disease, 3:85–87; Particulates, 8:65–66

Asbestosis, 3:86, 8:10
Ascorbic acid. *See* Vitamin C
Aspartame, 4:9
Aspiration, 6:4
Aspirin, 3:100, 108, 7:16, 30
  as anti-inflammatory drug, 7:28, 30
  dangers of, 7:30
  drug interactions with, 7:23, 30
  Reye's syndrome and, 2:20, 38, 53, 7:30
  side effects of, 7:48, 79
  uses of, 7:30
  See also Analgesics, 7:15–17

Assertiveness, 5:7, 12–13, 94. *See also* Communication, 5:22–23; Self-esteem, 5:88–89
Assertiveness training, 5:13
Association areas, 5:20, 21
Associative learning. *See* Conditioning
Asthma, 1:63, 3:6, 17–19, 18
  bronchodilators to treat, 7:34
  See also Lung, 1:62–63; Bronchitis, 2:17–18; Pneumonia, 2:72–73

Astigmatism, 3:116, 117
Ataxic cerebral palsy, 3:37
Atherosclerosis, 1:11, 12, 27, 3:19–20, 20, 68–69
  cholesterol and, 4:23
  See also Artery, 1:12; Arteriosclerosis, 3:15; Blood clot, 3:24; Heart disease, 3:69–72; Hypertension, 3:77–78; Stroke, 3:106–8; Risk factors, 4:94–95

Athletes
  diets for, 4:31
  drug abuse by, 7:52–53
Athlete's foot, 1:42, 90, 2:12, 3:57
  treating, 7:25
  See also Fungal infections, 2:38–39

Athletic footwear, 4:9–10, 96, 106
Atrial fibrillation, 3:70
Atrium (atria), 1:48
Atrophic vaginitis, 6:102
Attention deficit hyperactivity disorder (ADHD), 5:50–51
Attitudes, 5:13–14
  prejudice and, 5:72–74
  values and, 5:100–101
  See also Peer pressure, 5:67–68

Attraction, sexual, 6:87–88
Attributes, defining, 5:24
Atypical sexual behavior, 6:9
  pornography, 6:72–73
  sexual abuse, 6:87
  sexual fantasies, 6:89–90
Auditory nerve, 1:34
Aura of migraine, 3:88
Auricle (pinna), 1:33
Authoritarian leaders, 5:55
Autism, 5:14. *See also* Psychotherapy, 5:79–82
Autogenic training, 5:84, 99
Autoimmune disorder, 2:51, 77, 3:20, 112
  immunosuppressants to treat, 7:65
  silicone-gel implants and, 6:15
  See also Immune system, 1:52–55; Anemia, 3:11–12; Lupus erythematosus, 3:87; Mononucleosis, 3:38; Multiple sclerosis, 3:89–90

Automatic responses, coma and, 3:40
Automobile safety, 8:11–13
  defensive driving and, 8:13
  drinking and driving, 7:46–47, 8:12
  drugs and, 8:12
  equipment for, 8:78
  motor vehicle accidents and, 8:5, 11, 12

  safety features, 8:11–12
  traffic laws and, 8:12
  vehicle maintenance and, 8:12
  weather conditions and, 8:13
  See also Bicycle safety, 8:14; First aid kit, 8:39–40; Motorcycle safety, 8:58

Autonomic nervous system, 1:73, 5:15–16
  effects of, 5:15, 16
  emotions and, 5:42
  See also Adrenal glands, 1:6–7; Epinephrine, 1:38–39; Nervous system, 1:71–74; Central nervous system, 5:20–21

Autonomy versus shame and doubt, 5:35
Autopsy, 2:13, 9:29
Aversion therapy, 5:17
Avoidant personality disorder, 5:71
Avulsion, 8:101
Axons, 1:71, 74, 93
AZT (azidothymidine, zidovudine), 2:7, 7:29, 30, 31. *See also* AIDS, 2:4–8

Baby blues. *See* Postpartum depression
Bacillary dysentery, 2:31
Bacilli, 2:13, 15, 63
Bacitracin, 7:20
Back pain, 1:94
Back problems, 3:21–22, 21
  sports and, 4:102, 103
  See also Musculoskeletal system, 1:68–69; Spine, 1:94–95; Arthritis, 3:15–17

Bacteria, 2:63–64
  abscess caused by, 2:4
  anaerobic, 2:89–90
  culture, 2:9
  salmonella, 2:80, 80
  testing water for, 8:97
  tetanus, 2:89–90, 90
  types of, 2:13, 15

Bacterial contamination, 4:62
Bacterial food poisoning, 4:57–58
Bacterial infections, 2:13–15
  antibiotics for, 2:14, 64, 7:20–22
  cancer and, 3:30
  conjunctivitis caused by, 2:26
  croup, 2:28
  cystitis, 2:29
  defenses against, 2:14–15
  endocarditis, 2:34–35
  Legionnaires' disease, 2:55–56
  leprosy, 2:56–57

Lyme disease, 2:58–59
pelvic inflammatory disease after, 2:70
puerperal sepsis, 2:74
salmonella infections, 2:80
streptococcal infections, 2:86–87
sulfa drugs for, 7:96–97
tetanus, 2:89–90
tuberculosis, 2:94–95
whooping cough, 2:100
See also Diarrhea, 2:29–30; Immunization, 2:47–49; Microorganisms, 2:63–65; Food poisoning, 4:57–58; Antiseptics, 7:28–29
Bacterial meningitis, 2:61, 62
Bacterial pneumonia, 2:72, 73
Baking soda (sodium bicarbonate), 4:98
Balance, inner ear and, 1:34
Balance in weight training, 4:132
Baldness. *See* Hair loss
Ball-and-socket joints, 1:50, 56, *56*, 77, 87–88, *87*
Ballistic stretching, 4:109
Balloon angioplasty, 3:19
Barbiturates, 7:31–32, 87–88
side effects and risks of, 7:32
as sleeping pills, 7:90
See also Drug interaction, 7:47–48; Drug overdose, 7:48–49; Drug use and abuse, 7:55–57
Bard, Philip, 5:42
Bargaining stage of dying, 5:40
Barium enema, 3:39
Barium X ray, 3:40, 118
Barnard, Christiaan, 3:73
Barrier methods of contraception, 6:18, 22–24, 25, 26–27, 29
Basal cell carcinoma, 3:102, *103*
Basal cells, 1:89
Basal metabolic rate (BMR), 1:64–65, 4:15–16, 37–38, *37*
Baseline mammograms, 6:54
Basic health insurance, 9:16
Basic-level concepts, 5:24, *24*
Basic trust versus mistrust, 5:35
Batteries, solar, 8:84
B cells, 1:13, 53–54
BCG vaccine, 2:95
Bee stings, 8:16–17
Behavioral component of emotions, 5:42
Behavioral theories of personality, 5:69–70
Behaviorism, 5:76–77
Behavior modification, 5:16–18. *See also* Anxiety disorders, 5:10–12

Behavior therapy, 5:80
for hyperactivity, 5:51
Bends, 8:13–14, 99
Benign tumor, 3:29, 114
Benzene, 8:48
Benzidine, 8:48
Benzocaine, 7:43–44
Benzophenone, 7:97
Bereavement, 5:40–41
Beta-blocker, 3:69, 78, 89, 7:27, 32. *See also* Heart disease, 3:69–72; Hypertension, 3:77–78
Beta carotene, 4:10, 65, 116. *See also* Nutrients, 4:82–84; Vitamins, 4:121–22
Beta waves, 1:92
Beverages, 4:10–12, 123. *See also* Caffeine, 7:35–36
Bicarbonate, 1:76
Biceps muscles, 1:34–35, 67, *67*
Bicuspids (premolars), 1:99
Bicycle riding. *See* Cycling
Bicycle safety, 8:14
accidents and, 8:6, 14
equipment for, 8:14, 79
Bifocals, 3:117
Bile, 1:32, 42, 61, 100
Bile duct, 1:42
blockage of, 3:58, *58*
Bilirubin, excess of, 3:81, *81*
Binge eating, 4:34
Biodegradable solid waste, 8:86
Bioelectrical impedance, 4:14, 127
Bioequivalence of generic drug, 7:59, 60
Bioethics. *See* Medical ethics
Biofeedback, 3:94, 4:94, 5:18, 84, 99
Bioflavonoids, 4:118
Biological age, 9:13
Biological carcinogens, 3:33
Biological clock. *See* Circadian rhythm
Biological death, 1:28
Biological determinism, 5:63–64
Biologically based psychotherapy, 5:79, 81–82
Biological treatment of hazardous wastes, 8:48
Biological water pollutants, 8:95–96, *96*
Biopsy, 3:22–23, 26–27, 30, 38, 39, 77, 81
Biosphere, 8:14–15, *15*
effects of global warming on, 8:45, 46
as vast ecosystem, 8:29
See also Acid rain, 8:6–7; Air pollution, 8:9–10; Population growth, 8:70–72; Thermal

pollution, 8:91; Water pollution, 8:95–97
Biotin, 4:*116*, 117, *121*
Bipolar disorder, 5:18–19, 34, 39. *See also* Depression, 5:32–34; Self-esteem, 5:88–89; Suicide, 5:99–100; Antidepressants, 7:23–24
Birth. *See* Childbirth
Birth centers, 6:65
Birth-control pill, 6:9–11, 25. *See also* Contraception, 6:24–26; Female reproductive system, 6:33–34; Infertility, 6:50–51; Ovulation, 6:68; Pregnancy, 6:74–76; Sex hormones, 6:84–85
Birth defects, 6:4, 11–12
Down syndrome, 3:49–50
fetal alcohol syndrome and, 7:58–59
risk factors for, 6:11, 12
sedative use during pregnancy and, 7:88
sickle cell anemia, 3:102
Tay-Sachs disease, 3:110
See also Rubella, 2:78–79; Fetus, 6:37–38; Genetics, 6:40–42; Genetic screening, 6:42–44; Radiation, 8:72–74
Bisexuality, 6:12–13, 45, 47. *See also* Gender identity, 6:38–40
Bites and stings, 8:15–18
animal, 8:16, 17, 55
insect, 8:16–17, 55
insect repellent to prevent, 7:67–68
Lyme disease and, 2:58–59
rabies and, 2:75
Rocky Mountain spotted fever and, 2:78
tick, 2:91
See also Tetanus, 2:89–90; Shock, 3:101; First aid kit, 8:39–40
Black Death (bubonic plague), 2:36, 71
Blackheads, 3:4, *4*
Black lung disease, 3:86, *86*
Black-market adoptions, 6:6
Bladder, 1:101
inflammation of, 2:29
Bladder problems, 3:80, 82
Bleeding, 8:18–19
cerebral hemorrhage, 3:107
controlling, 8:18, 19, 39
external, 8:18
hemophilia and, 3:74–75
internal, 3:114, 8:18–19
iron-deficiency anemia caused by, 3:11
nosebleeds, 3:91–92

peptic ulcers as cause of, 3:114
and pressure point technique, 8:18, *18*
wound first aid, 8:18, 101
See also Blood pressure, 1:14–16; Shock, 3:101; Injuries, 8:55–56
Blended family, 5:44
Blindness
  color, 1:23
  night, 3:54
Blind studies, 7:37
Blisters, 3:23–24, 51, 57
  cold sore, 2:23
  of herpes infection, 2:44
  of impetigo, 2:49–50, 3:23
  sports and, 4:103
  from sunburn, 8:88–89
  See also Eczema, 3:51
Blizzards, 8:101
Blood, 1:12–14, *13*
  heart and circulation of, 1:47–49
  and inflammatory response, 1:53
  in urine, 1:100
  See also Blood pressure, 1:14–16; Blood test, 1:16; Blood type, 1:17; Immune system, 1:52–55; AIDS, 2:4–8; HIV, 2:45–46; Anemia, 3:11–12; Blood clot, 3:24; Hemophilia, 3:74–75; Leukemia, 3:83–84; Bleeding, 8:18–19
Blood alcohol level (BAL), 7:6, 7, 33–34
  effects of, 7:*33*, 34
  factors affecting, 7:33–34
  legal intoxication defined, 7:9, 33, 46, 68
  measuring, 7:34
  See also Social drinking, 7:92–93
Blood bank, 1:14. *See also* Blood test, 1:16; Blood type, 1:17; Rh factor, 6:82
Blood blisters, 3:23
Blood cells, 1:12–13, *13*
  red. *See* Red blood cells (erythrocytes)
  white. *See* White blood cells (leukocytes)
Blood clot, 1:13, 3:24, *24*
  aneurysm forming, 3:14
  anticoagulants to prevent abnormal, 7:23
  in coronary artery, 3:68, *68*, 69
  in hemorrhoid, 3:75
  pulmonary embolism caused by, 3:86
  stroke caused by, 3:106–7, *107*
  See also Circulatory system, 1:25–27; Arteriosclerosis, 3:15;

Atherosclerosis, 3:19–20; Cardiovascular disease, 3:34; Heart disease, 3:69–72; Varicose vein, 3:115–16
Blood poisoning, 3:24–25, 101
Blood pressure, 1:14–16, 102
  antihypertensives to lower, 7:27
  normal, 3:77
  See also Heart, 1:47–49, Atherosclerosis, 3:19–20; Hypertension, 3:77–78
Blood proteins, 1:61, 4:91
Blood sugar level, 4:67
Blood test, 1:16
  for anemia, 3:11
  See also Blood type, 1:17; Microorganisms, 2:63–65
Blood transfusion, 3:25, 75
  blood bank and, 1:14
  blood type and, 1:17
  HIV transmission through, 2:5, 46
  See also Blood, 1:12–14; AIDS, 2:4–8; Immunity, 2:47
Blood type, 1:17
  Rh factor and, 6:82
  See also Blood transfusion, 3:25
Blood vessel constrictors, 7:58
Boating safety, 8:99
Body building, 4:12–13. *See also* Anaerobic exercise, 4:7; Strength exercise, 4:108–9; Weight training, 4:132–33; Steroids, 7:94–95
Body clock. *See* Circadian rhythm
Body composition, 4:13–14
  body building and changing, 4:13
  fitness and, 4:49
  managing, 4:131
  measuring, 4:14
  weight assessment and, 4:124
  See also Diets, 4:30–32; Eating disorders, 4:33–34; Obesity, 4:85–86
Body fat, 4:14–15
  body composition and, 4:13
  food energy and, 4:35–36
  See also Atherosclerosis, 3:19–20; Heart disease, 3:69–72; Cholesterol, 4:23–24; Fats, oils, and sweets group, 4:46–47; Risk factors, 4:94–95
Body image, 4:33, 124
  anorexia and, 4:33, 5:8
Body language, 5:19, 22. *See also* Communication, 5:22–23
Body lice, 2:57
Body-mass index (BMI), 4:14, 87, 126, *126*

Body metabolism, 4:15–17
  epilepsy and, 3:54
  fasting and, 4:43–44
  measuring, 4:15–16
  obesity and, 4:85
  protein and, 4:91
  See also Digestion, 4:32–33; Metabolism, 1:64–65; Nutrients, 4:82–84
Body of sternum, 1:24
Body temperature, 1:22, 53, 89, 8:19
  basal metabolic rate and, 4:16
  fever and, 2:37–38
  heatstroke and, 8:49
  hypothermia and, 8:54–55
  measuring, 8:19, 57
  sports and heat problems, 4:101–2
Body types, 4:*14*
Boil, 1:90, 2:15–16. *See also* Abscess, 2:4; Bacterial infections, 2:13–15
Bomb calorimeter, 4:20
Bone(s), 1:17–18
  carpal, 1:46, 3:35
  disorders of, 1:18
  of elbow, 1:34–35, *35*
  facial, 1:91
  of foot, 1:41, *41*
  of hand, 1:46, 47, 3:35
  in musculoskeletal system, 1:68–69, *68*
  osteomyelitis of, 2:68
  osteoporosis and, 3:93
  pelvic, 1:77, *77*
  skull, 1:91
  structure of, 1:*18*
  See also Bone marrow, 1:18–19; Arthritis, 3:15–17
Bone fracture, 3:93, *118*, 8:41–43, *42*
Bone graft, 3:97
Bone marrow, 1:18–19
  transplantation of, 1:19, 3:84, 113
  See also Anemia, 3:11–12; Leukemia, 3:83–84
Bone strength, 4:49
Booster shots, 2:48
Bottled water, 8:98
Bottle-feeding, 6:14
Botulism, 2:14, 94, 4:52, 57–58, 63
Bowel movements, 3:41–42, 80
  diarrhea and, 2:29–30
Braces. *See* Orthodontic devices
Bradycardia, 8:72
Braille, 8:4
Brain, 1:19–21, *20*
  alcohol abuse and effect on, 7:9
  Alzheimer's disease and, 3:9
  brain waves during sleep, 1:91–92

cerebral palsy and, 3:36–37
dreams and, 5:38–39
electroencephalogram of, 3:52
encephalitis infection of, 2:34
epilepsy and electrical function
of, 3:53–54
functions of, 5:20, *21*
growth of, 1:43–44
interpretation of pain, 3:*94*
and nervous system, 1:72
organic disorders of, 5:66
perception and, 5:68
Reye's syndrome and, 3:100
stroke and, 3:106–8
Tay-Sachs disease and, 3:110
See also Hypothalamus, 1:52;
Neuron, 1:74–75; Parkinson's
disease, 3:95–96
Brain damage, effects of, 3:36, 40–41
Brain death, 1:28
Brain stem, 1:19, 5:20
Brain tumor, 1:74, 3:25–26, *26*, 43,
44. *See also* Cancer, 3:29–32
Bran, 4:17
Brand-name drugs, 7:52, 59, 60
Bravery, 5:46
Breads and cereals group, 4:17–18,
50, 60, 64, *64*
starch and, 4:106–7
See also Exchange system,
4:38–39; Five food groups system, 4:50–51; Food pyramid
system, 4:60–61; Four food
groups system, 4:64–65
Breaking of the waters, 6:7
Breast, 6:13–14, *13*, 34
examination by gynecologist,
6:45
mammogram of, 6:45, 54–55, *54*
mastectomy, 6:56–57, *57*
milk production in, 4:18–19,
6:13, 14, *14*
See also Breast cancer, 3:26–28;
Breast implants, 6:15
Breast cancer, 3:26–28, *30*
biopsy for, 3:26–27
birth-control pills and, 6:10, 11
early detection of, 6:15–17,
54–55
mastectomy for, 6:56–57, *57*
See also Tumor, 3:114; Mammogram, 6:54–55
Breast examination, clinical, 3:26
Breast-feeding, 1:54, 4:18, 6:14
breast milk for, 4:18–19
See also Immune system, 1:52–55
Breast implants, 3:97, 6:15, *15*
breast self-examination and,
6:16–17

See also Autoimmune disorder,
3:20; Breast cancer, 3:26–28;
Plastic surgery, 3:97; Food and
Drug Administration, 7:59
Breast milk, 4:18, 6:13, 14, *14*. *See
also* Antibody, 2:10; Breast, 6:13–14
Breast self-examination, 6:14, 15–17,
16. *See also* Breast cancer, 3:26–28;
Mammogram, 6:54–55
Breathalyzer test, 7:34, 55
Breathing cycle, 1:84
Breathing difficulties, 2:16–17,
3:17–18, *53*, 79
asthma and, 3:17–19
bronchitis and, 2:17–18
croup and, 2:27–28
emphysema and, 3:53
hyperventilation and, 3:79
pleurisy and, 3:98
pneumonia and, 2:72–73
See also Respiratory system,
1:84–86; Heart disease,
3:69–72
Breathing exercises, 4:94
Bridges (partial dentures), 3:46
Broad-spectrum antibiotics, 2:9, 7:21
Bronchi, 1:63, 84
Bronchial asthma. *See* Asthma
Bronchial tubes, 1:62, 84
Bronchioles, 1:63, 84
Bronchitis, 1:85, 2:17–18, *18*
asthma and, 3:18
chronic, 1:63
See also Breathing difficulties,
2:16–17; Cough, 2:27; Infec-
tion, 2:50–51; Inflammation,
2:51–52; Emphysema, 3:53;
Bronchodilator, 7:34–35
Bronchodilator, 2:18, 3:18, 7:34–35.
See also Respiratory system,
1:84–86; Bronchitis, 2:17–18;
Asthma, 3:17–19; Corticosteroids,
7:40
Brown rice, 4:18
Brown sugar, 4:111
Bruises, 1:27, 4:103, 8:101
Bruxism, 3:110
Bubonic plague, 2:36, 71
Bulimia, 4:33, 34, 5:8
Bulk-forming laxatives, 7:69
Bulking agents, 7:24
Bunions, 1:42, 3:57
Burial of hazardous waste, 8:48, 49
Burn center, 8:32
Burns, 8:5, 20–21, 56
classifying, 8:20, *20*
from clothing fires, 8:37
first aid for, 8:20–21
lightning-caused, 8:100

sun damage, 8:88–89
See also Shock, 3:101; Electric
shock, 8:31; Fire safety,
8:36–37
Bursa, 1:58, 88, 3:28, *28*, 57
Bursitis, 1:59, 88, 3:28
Butterfat, 4:78
Bypass surgery, 3:73

Caffeine, 4:11, 12, 7:35–36, *35*, 85,
96
in look-alike drugs, 7:70
withdrawal symptoms from,
7:35, 101
See also Antihistamines and decongestants, 7:25–27; Diet
pills, 7:43–44; Diuretic(s),
7:44–45
Calcaneus, 1:41
Calcitonin, 1:*51*, 97
Calcium, 4:19–20, 31, 79, *80*, 114
in bone, osteoporosis and, 3:93
regulation of level of, 1:97
See also Minerals, 4:79–81; Vitamins, 4:121–22
Calcium-channel blockers, 7:27
Calcium deficiency, 4:19–20
Calcium phosphate, 4:19
Calcium sorbate, 4:52
Calculus (tartar), 1:29, 3:62, 7:100
Calendar method of family planning,
6:66
Calluses, 1:42
Calorie(s), 4:20–21
diet and supply of, 4:30
empty, 4:70, 97
energy-balance equation,
4:20–21, 36, 131
in fats, 4:45
junk food and, 4:70–71
measuring food energy by, 4:36
requirements for energy, 4:37–38,
37
to support basal metabolism,
4:15–16
weight-gain strategy and, 4:128
weight-loss strategy and, 4:129
weight management and, 4:131
See also Metabolism, 1:64–65;
Body metabolism, 4:15–17
Cancer, 3:29–32, *30*
anticancer drugs and, 7:22–23
brain tumor, 3:25–26
breast cancer, 3:26–28
cancers of the sex organs,
6:17–18
carcinogens and, 3:33
chemotherapy for, 3:31, 37

colorectal cancer, 3:40
Hodgkin's disease, 3:77
Kaposi's sarcoma, 3:81–82
leukemia, 3:83–84
lung cancer, 3:85
lymphatic system and spread of,
    1:64
lymphoma, 3:87
macrobiotic diet and, 4:73
radiation therapy for, 3:99
skin, 3:102–3
smokeless tobacco and, 7:36
smoking and, 7:90–91
warning signs, 3:30
See also Biopsy, 3:22–23; Surgery,
    3:108–9; Tumor, 3:114
Cancer cells, 3:29
Cancer immunotherapy, 3:31–32, 80
Cancer quackery, 9:37
Cancers of the sex organs, 6:17–18
detection of, 6:45, 69, 98–99
See also Cancer, 3:29–32;
    Chemotherapy, 3:37; Radiation
    therapy, 3:99; Female repro-
    ductive system, 6:33–34; Male
    reproductive system, 6:52–54;
    STDs, 6:94–95
Candida albicans, 2:19, 6:102
Candida infections, 2:19
antibiotic use and, 7:21
Candidiasis, 6:101, 102
treating, 7:25
Canines (cuspids), 1:99
Canker sore, 3:32. See also Cold sore,
    2:23; Herpes infections, 2:44–45
Cannabis sativa, 7:71
Canning, 4:59
Cannon, Walter, 5:42
Cannon-Bard theory of emotion,
    5:42, 43
Cannula, 6:4
Capillary(ies), 1:21–22, 25, 26
Capillary bleeding, 8:18
Capsules, 7:83
Captopril, 7:27
Carbohydrates, 4:21–22, 83, 83
breads and cereals group,
    4:17–18
complex, 4:21, 22, 106–7
craving for foods high in, 4:54
energy from, 4:35–36
fiber, 4:47–48
fruits and vegetables group,
    4:65–66
simple, 4:21, 22, 106
starch, 4:106–7
sugar, 4:110–11
See also Glucose, 4:66–67; Nutri-
    ents, 4:82–84

Carbon dioxide, 8:21
air pollution caused by, 8:9
in blood, 3:79
energy conservation and reduc-
    tion of, 8:34
greenhouse effect and, 8:45–46,
    45
See also Biosphere, 8:14–15
Carbon dioxide–oxygen exchange,
    1:12, 26, 62, 63, 84
Carbon monoxide in tobacco smoke,
    7:91, 98
Carbon monoxide poisoning,
    8:21–22, 91
Carbon tetrachloride, 8:48
Carbuncle, 2:15, 16
Carcinogens, 3:30, 33, 6:64
asbestos, 8:10–11
in tobacco, 7:98
Carcinoma, 3:29–30, 102, 103
Cardiac asthma, 3:17. See also Heart
    attack, 3:68–69
Cardiac (heart) surgery, 3:73–74,
    109
Cardiac muscle, 1:67
Cardiologists, 9:33
Cardiomyopathy, 3:71
Cardiopulmonary resuscitation. See
    CPR
Cardiovascular disease, 3:34
aneurysm, 3:13–14
arteriosclerosis, 3:15
atherosclerosis, 3:19–20
endocarditis, 2:34–35
heart attack, 3:68–69
heart disease, 3:69–72
rheumatic fever, 2:77–78
smoking and, 7:91
See also Circulatory system,
    1:25–27; Heart, 1:47–49;
    Blood clot, 3:24; Heart mur-
    mur, 3:72–73; Heart surgery,
    3:73–74; Hypertension,
    3:77–78
Cardiovascular endurance, 4:34, 35,
    49
Cardiovascular fitness, 4:4, 5, 6, 68,
    100
Cardiovascular system. See Circula-
    tory system
Caries, dental, 1:99, 3:44, 45
Carotid arteries, 1:70
taking pulse in, 8:72
Carpal bones, 1:46, 3:35
Carpal tunnel syndrome, 1:46–47,
    3:34–35. See also Hand, 1:46–47
Car pools, 8:34
Carriers, 2:25
Car seats, 8:12, 78

Cartilage, 1:27, 56
of elbow, 1:35
in hip joint, 1:50
of knee, 1:58
Catabolism, 1:64, 4:15
Catalysts, enzymes as, 1:37
Cataracts, 3:35–36, 35
ozone-layer depletion and in-
    crease in, 8:65
See also Eye, 1:39–41; Eye dis-
    orders, 3:54–55; Eye tests, 3:55
CAT scan, 2:34, 3:26, 36. See also
    Magnetic resonance imaging (MRI),
    3:88; X-ray examination, 3:117–18
Cavity, dental, 3:44, 45
Cecum, 1:11
Celiac disease, diet for, 4:32
Cell(s), 1:22–23
disorders of, 1:23
division, 1:23, 6:30, 36, 40
structure of, 1:22, 23
types of, 1:22, 22
See also Tissue, 1:98; Genetics,
    6:40–42; specific types of cells
Cell body of neuron, 1:74
Cementum, 1:99
Centers for Disease Control (CDC),
    2:53, 3:38, 9:8–9, 9
Central nervous system, 1:71,
    5:20–21
damage to, 5:21
functions of brain, 1:19–21,
    5:20, 21
intoxication and, 7:9, 68
narcotics' effect on, 7:77
spinal cord and, 1:93–94
See also Nervous system,
    1:71–74; Autonomic nervous
    system, 5:15–16; Emotion,
    5:42–44; Perception, 5:68;
    Personality(ies), 5:69–70
Cephalosporins, 7:21
Cereals, 4:17
Cerebellum, 1:21, 5:20. See also
    Pineal gland, 1:79; Pituitary gland,
    1:79–80
Cerebral cortex, 1:21, 5:20, 21, 62
Cerebral embolism, 3:106–7, 107
Cerebral hemorrhage, 3:107
Cerebral palsy, 3:36–37
Cerebral thrombosis, 3:106, 107
Cerebrovascular accident (CVA). See
    Stroke
Cerebrum, 1:21, 5:20
Cervical cancer, Pap test to detect,
    6:17, 69
Cervical cap, 6:18, 25
Cervical dysplasia, 6:69
Cervical mucus, 6:66, 68

Cervical vertebrae, 1:70, *70, 94*
Cervix, **1:**83, 6:33
  dilation of, during childbirth, 6:20
Cesarean section, 6:19, *19*
  for multiple births, 6:63
  placenta previa and, 6:72
  See also Apgar test, 6:8–9; Female
    reproductive system, 6:33–34;
    Fetus, 6:37–38; Miscarriage,
    6:61–62; Prenatal care, 6:78
Cestode. *See* Tapeworm
Chafing, 4:103
Chancre, **2:**88
Charismatic leadership, **5:**55
Chemical barrier method of contra-
  ception, 6:24
Chemical carcinogens, 3:33
Chemical preservation, 4:52, 59–60,
  63
Chemicals, agricultural, 4:6–7, 86,
  8:7. *See also* Toxic substances,
  8:91–92
Chemical treatment of hazardous
  wastes, 8:48
Chemotherapy, 3:31, 37, 7:22. *See
  also* Cancer, 3:29–32; Radiation
  therapy, 3:99; Surgery, 3:108–9
Chernobyl nuclear power plant, 8:62
Chest, 1:23–24, *24*
  diaphragm (muscle) in, 1:30
Chest compressions, 8:24, *25*
Chest X ray, **2:**95
  of pneumonia, 2:72
Chewing tobacco and snuff, 7:36. *See
  also* Cancer, 3:29–32; Dental
  problems, 3:44–45
Chicken pox, 1:90, 2:19–20
  blisters of, 3:23
  See also Shingles, 2:83–84; Viral
    infections, 2:97–98; Reye's syn-
    drome, 3:100
Child abuse, 5:6, 8:22–23, 92
  incest and, 6:49–50
  among teenage parents, 6:98
  See also Spouse abuse, 8:86
Childbed fever. *See* Puerperal sepsis
Childbirth, 6:20–21
  Apgar test for newborns, 6:8–9, *8*
  beginning of, 6:20, *75*
  breaking of the waters, 6:7
  cesarean section, 6:19, *19*
  medical ethics involving,
    9:21–22
  multiple births, 6:36, 62–63
  natural, 6:20, 21, 64–65
  placenta in, 6:71–72
  postpartum depression after,
    6:73–74
  premature baby and, 6:76–77

preparing for, 6:21
stages of labor, 6:20–21, 64
for teenagers, 6:98
umbilical cord in, 6:101
See also Female reproductive
  system, 6:33–34
Child development, 1:24–25
  adolescence, 1:5–6
Child pornography, 6:73
Childproof caps, 8:68
Childproofing, 8:69
Children
  accidents common among, 8:5,
    6, 53
  adoption of, 6:6–7
  of alcoholics, 7:11–12
  developing self-esteem in, 5:89
  developmental psychology and,
    5:34–36
  divorce and, 5:37
  in dysfunctional family, 5:45
  gender identity of, 6:39
  incest and, 6:49–50
  lead poisoning in, 8:56, 91
  malnutrition among, 4:74–75
  parenthood and, 6:69–71
  poisonings among, 8:5, 6, 68, 69
  prenatal drug exposure of. *See*
    Pregnancy
  violence in the media and, 8:93
Children and youth services department, 8:23
Chinese restaurant syndrome, 4:82
Chiropractic, 9:4, 5–6
Chiropractor, 9:5–6
Chlamydia, 6:*94*
Chlamydial infections, 2:20–21, *21,*
  67. *See also* Pelvic inflammatory
  disease (PID), 2:70–71; Sexually
  transmitted diseases (STDs), 2:82
Chlamydia trachomatis, 2:20, *21*
Chloride, 4:79–80
Chlorinated hydrocarbons, water pol-
  luted with, 8:96, *96*
Chlorination, 8:97
Chlorofluorocarbons (CFCs), 8:10,
  64–65
Chloroquine, 2:60
Choking, 1:96, 8:24, 39
  Heimlich maneuver to stop, 8:24,
    39, 50–51, *50*
  See also CPR, 8:24–25
Cholera, 2:22–23, 25. *See also* Epi-
  demic, 2:36; Toxin, 2:94
Cholesterol, 1:61, 3:19, *20,* 58, *71,*
  4:5, 23–24, *24,* 45, 47, 77. *See also*
  Body fat, 4:14–15; Fast food, 4:43;
  Food labeling, 4:56–57; Meats,
  eggs, and legumes group, 4:75–77;

Obesity, 4:85–86; Risk factors,
  4:94–95
Chorionic villi, 6:71
Chorionic villus sampling, 6:43–44,
  78
  ultrasound during, 6:100
Chromium, 4:*80,* 81
Chromosomes, 1:22, 23, 6:36, 40, *41,*
  63
  abnormalities of, 6:11
  extra, 3:49, *50*
  homologous, 6:40
  X and Y, 6:40, 42
Chronic bronchitis, 2:17–18
Chronic diarrhea, 2:30
Chronic fatigue syndrome (CFS),
  3:38. *See also* Immune system,
  1:52–55; Mononucleosis, 2:65
Chronic glaucoma, 3:60
Chronic hepatitis, 2:43
Chronic lymphocytic leukemia
  (CLL), 3:*84*
Chronic myeloid leukemia (CML),
  3:*84*
Chronic obstructive lung disease
  (COLD), 2:18
Chronic obstructive pulmonary dis-
  ease (COPD), 2:18
Chronic renal failure, 3:82–83
Chronic shyness, 5:91
Chronic sinusitis, 2:84
Chronological age, 9:13
Cigarette smoke, respiratory prob-
  lems and, 1:85–86, 7:91
Cilia, 1:63, 84, 7:91
  of lungs, 8:65
Circadian rhythm, 1:79, 5:22. *See
  also* Sleep problems, 5:93–94
Circuit training, 4:132
Circulatory system, 1:25–27, *26*
  arteries in, 1:12
  capillaries in, 1:21–22
  effect of alcohol abuse on, 7:9
  gangrene and lack of circulation,
    3:59
  pulmonary circulation, 1:26
  systemic circulation, 1:26
  veins in, 1:102
  See also Atherosclerosis, 3:19–20;
    Cardiovascular disease, 3:34;
    Hypertension, 3:77–78; Vari-
    cose vein, 3:115–16; Aerobic
    exercise, 4:4–6
Circumcision, 6:21–22, *22,* 54. *See
  also* Cancers of the sex organs,
  6:17–18; Male reproductive system,
  6:52–54
Cirrhosis, 1:61–62, 3:38–39, *39. See
  also* Liver, 1:60–62; Hepatitis,

2:42–43; Jaundice, 3:81; Peritonitis, 3:97; Alcoholism, 7:12–14
Citizen action groups against drunk driving, 7:46–47
Classical conditioning, 5:25–26, 25, 56
Clavicle, 1:87–88
Clean Air Acts, 8:10, 66
Clean-catch specimen, 1:100
Cleanliness, food preparation and, 4:62
Cleft lip, 6:11, 11
Cleft palate, 1:91
Climate, global warming and, 8:45–46
Climaxing. See Orgasm
Clinic, 9:6–7
    group medical care at, 9:13
Clinical Center (NIH), 9:9
Clinical death, 1:28
Clinical dietitians, 9:26
Clinical disease stage of infection, 2:50
Clinical drug trials, 7:37
    placebos used in, 7:82
Clinical psychology, 5:77
Clitoris, 1:83, 6:33
Closed adoption, 6:6
Closed captioning, 8:4
Closed fracture, 8:41
Clostridium botulinum, 4:57
Clostridium perfringens, 4:57
Clot, blood. See Blood clot
Clotting factors, 7:23
Clubfoot, 6:12
Cluster headaches, 3:66
Coal, 8:40
Cocaine, 7:17, 37–38, 96
    crack, 7:38, 53–54
    effects of, 7:38
    risks of, 7:38
    use of, 7:37–38
    See also AIDS, 2:4–8; Addiction, 7:4–5; Drug overdose, 7:48–49; Drug rehabilitation, 7:49–50; Drugs and the law, 7:53–54; Drug use and abuse, 7:55–57; Injection, 7:67; Withdrawal syndrome, 7:100–101
Cocaine hydrochloride, 7:37–38
Cocci, 2:13, 15, 63
Coccyx, 1:94
Cochlea, 1:33, 34, 3:67, 67
Codeine, 7:16, 16, 41, 77, 79
Codependency, 5:83, 7:39–40
Coenzyme, 1:38
Coffee, 4:12
Cognitive aspect of emotion, 5:42
Cognitive consistency, theory of, 5:14

Cognitive development, 5:34–35, 57
Cognitive dissonance, 5:14
Cognitive labeling theory of emotion, 5:43, 43
Cognitive learning, 5:57
Cognitive therapy, 5:80
Cohabitation, 6:56, 56
Cold method of food preservation, 4:59
Cold sore, 1:65, 2:23, 44
Cold-weather emergencies, 8:101
Colectomy, 3:40
Coliform bacteria, testing water for, 8:97
Colitis, 2:30, 3:39
Collagen, 1:17, 27, 28, 86
Collar-button abscess, 2:4
Colon, 1:32, 39, 81
    diverticulitis in, 3:49
    pinworms in, 2:69
Color blindness, 1:23
Colorectal cancer, 3:40. See also Colitis, 3:39; Tumor, 3:114; Fats, 4:45–46; Fiber, 4:47–48
Coloring agents, 4:53
Color vision deficiency, 3:54
Colostomy, 3:40
Colostrum, 4:19, 6:14
Coma, 3:40–41. See also Brain, 1:19–21; Brain tumor, 3:25–26; Epilepsy, 3:53–54; Stroke, 3:106–8; Medical ethics, 9:21–22
Combat fatigue. See Post-traumatic stress disorder (PTSD)
Coming. See Orgasm
Common cold, 1:76, 85, 2:23–24
    croup and, 2:28
    treatment for, 7:25–27
    See also Bronchitis, 2:17–18; Cough, 2:27; Laryngitis, 2:54–55; Sinusitis, 2:84–85
Common wart, 2:99
Communicable diseases, 2:24–26
    epidemics of, 2:36
    influenza, 2:52–53
    prevention of, 2:25, 26
    sexually transmitted diseases (STDs), 2:82
    spread of, 2:25, 8:80
    See also Immune system, 1:52–55; Antibiotic treatment, 2:8–10; Immunization, 2:47–49; Infection, 2:50–51; Microorganisms, 2:63–65
Communication, 5:22–23
    assertiveness, 5:12–13
    body language, 5:19
    effective, 5:23
    elements and types of, 5:22

See also Attitudes, 5:13–14; Conflict resolution, 5:27–28; Emotion, 5:42–44; Relationships, 5:82–83; Social skills, 5:94–95
Community crisis centers, 5:100
Community psychiatry, 5:75
Companionate love, 5:59
Competition, sibling rivalry and, 5:92
Competition theory of prejudice, 5:73
Complementary proteins, 4:76
Complete blood count (CBC), 1:16
Complete proteins, 4:76, 90
Complex carbohydrates, 4:21, 22, 106–7
Compliance, 5:13, 28–29
Composting, 8:75
Compound fracture, 8:41, 42
Compression of injured area, 8:76, 77
Compromises, 5:27, 28
Compulsions, 5:11
Compulsive personality disorder, 5:71
Computerized axial tomography. See CAT scan
Conception. See Fertilization
Concepts, 5:23–25
    learning, 5:24–25
    levels of, 5:24, 24
Concrete operational stage, 5:35
Conditioned reflex, 1:82
Conditioning, 5:25–27, 56
    in behavior modification, 5:16–18
    behavior therapy using, 5:80
    classical, 5:25–26, 25, 56
    operant, 5:25, 26–27, 56
    See also Learning, 5:56–57
Condom, 6:22–24, 25
    acquiring, 6:24
    advantages and disadvantages of, 6:22–23
    correct use of, 6:23
    prevention of disease with, 2:7, 21, 40, 6:83, 95
    for women, 6:24
    See also AIDS, 2:4–8; Herpes, genital, 2:44; Female reproductive system, 6:33–34; Male reproductive system, 6:52–54
Conductive deafness, 3:66–67
Cones, 1:40
Confidence, 5:88
Conflict between values, 5:100–101
Conflict resolution, 5:27–28. See also Anger, 5:7–8; Communication, 5:22–23; Relationships, 5:82–83; Stress, 5:95–98

Conformity, 5:28–29
  with peers, 5:67–68
  See also Attitudes, 5:13–14;
    Prosocial behavior, 5:74
Congenital cataracts, 3:35
Congenital heart disease, 3:72
Congenital syphilis, 2:88
Congestive heart failure, 3:17, 34, 68,
  70, 71–72
Conjunctiva, 2:26, 27
Conjunctivitis, 2:21, 26–27. *See also*
  Chlamydial infections, 2:20–21;
  Gonorrhea, 2:41–42
Connecting neurons, 1:72, 74, 93
Connective tissue, 1:27–28, 98
  lupus and, 3:87
  tendinitis, 3:111–12
  See also Arthritis, 3:15–17;
    Sports injuries, 4:102–5
Consciousness, 5:62–63
Consent, informed, 9:29
Conservation
  energy, 8:33–34, *34*, 40–41
  environmental organizations and,
    8:35, 90
  water, 8:94–95
Constipation, 3:41–42, 49, 75
  fiber and, 4:47–48
  laxatives to treat, 7:69–70
Consumption. *See* Tuberculosis
Contact dermatitis, 2:76, *76*, 3:6
Contact lenses, 3:117
Contact poisoning, 8:67, 70
Contamination of food, 4:62–63
Contentment, 5:48
Contraception, 6:24–26
  barrier methods of, 6:18, 22–24,
    25, 26–27, 29
  birth-control pill, 6:9–11
  cervical cap, 6:18
  choosing method of, 6:25–26, *25*
  condom, 6:22–24
  contraceptive implant, 6:26
  contraceptive sponge, 6:26–27
  diaphragm, 6:29
  hormonal methods of, 6:24, *25*
  IUD, 6:51–52
  methods under research, 6:26
  natural family planning, 6:66
  population control and, 8:71
  responsible sexual intercourse
    and, 6:91
  risk factors, 6:25
  sterilization, 6:96–97
  teenage pregnancy and, 6:97
  See also Female reproductive sys-
    tem, 6:33–34; Fertilization,
    6:35–37; Male reproductive
    system, 6:52–54; Safer sex,

6:82–83; Sex hormones,
    6:84–85
Contraceptive implant, 6:25, 26,
  7:83. *See also* Menstruation,
  6:59–61; Sex hormones, 6:84–85
Contraceptive sponge, 6:25, 26–27
Contract-relax stretching, 4:109–10,
  109
Control group, 7:37, 82
Controlled Substance Act, 7:43
Controlled substances, 7:53–54
Contusion, 8:101
Convalescence, 3:109
Conventional level of moral develop-
  ment, 5:36
Conversion disorder, 5:79
Convulsions, epilepsy and, 3:53, 54
Cooking vegetables, 4:65–66
Coping skills, 5:29–30
  assertiveness and, 5:12–13
  in dying and bereavement, 5:41
  for managing anger, 5:7–8
  relaxation training and, 5:84
  for stress, 5:29–30, 97–98
  See also Conflict resolution,
    5:27–28; Friendship, 5:46–47;
    Self-efficacy, 5:88
Copper, 4:80, 81
Coral, stings from, 8:17–18
Cornea, 1:39
  vision problems and, 3:116, *116*
Corns, 1:42, 3:57
Coronary artery bypass surgery,
  3:19–20, 69, 73
Coronary artery disease, 3:34, 68, *68*,
  69, 70
Coronary care units, 9:20
Coroner, 2:13
Corrosives, poisoning by, 8:67, 68
Cortex (hair), 1:45
Corticosteroids, 7:28, 40, 94
Cosmetic surgery, 3:97
Cough, 2:27
  bronchitis and persistent dry,
    2:17, 18
  croup, 2:27–28
  whooping, 2:100
  See also Common cold, 2:23–24;
    Influenza, 2:52–53
Cough medicine, 7:41, 73
Cough suppressants, 7:41
Counseling psychology, 5:77
Counselors, 9:36
  genetic, 9:12
Cowper's glands, 6:53
Cow's milk, sensitivity to, 4:54
CPR, 3:69, 8:24–25, *25*
  electric shock and, 8:31
  as emergency first aid, 8:38

See also Accidents, 8:5–6;
    Drowning, 8:26–27; Emer-
    gency care services, 8:32–33;
    First aid, 8:38–39; Heimlich
    maneuver, 8:50–51
Crack (cocaine), 7:38, 53–54
Cramps, 1:67, 4:103
  swimming and muscle cramping,
    8:98
Cranial bones, 1:91
Cranial cavity, 1:91
Craving, food, 4:54–55
Cream, 4:78
Creativity, 5:30. *See also* Self-
  actualization, 5:87
Cretinism, 1:97
Crib death. *See* Sudden infant death
  syndrome (SIDS)
Crime
  drugs and, 7:53, 54
  violent, 8:92–93
Crisis intervention, 5:31
  for post-traumatic stress dis-
    orders, 5:72
  suicide prevention, 5:100
Crohn's disease, 3:39
Cross-country ski machines, 4:41
Cross-dressing, 6:99, 100
Cross training, 4:24–25. *See also* Aer-
  obic exercise, 4:4–6; Exercise,
  4:39–40; Fitness, 4:48–49; Fitness
  training, 4:49–50; Sports and fit-
  ness, 4:99–101; Weight training,
  4:132–33
Croup, 2:27–28
Crown of tooth, 1:99
Cryosurgery, 3:103
Crystals in urine, 1:100
C-section. *See* Cesarean section
CT scan. *See* CAT scan
Culture, 2:28–29
  bacteria grown in, 2:9, *28*
  blood, 1:16
  throat, 2:28–29, 78, 86
Cultured milk products, 4:78
Culture medium, 2:29
Culture (social)
  attitudes learned from, 5:13
  emotional development and, 5:43
  masturbation and, 6:57
  values and, 5:100
Cunnilingus, 6:67
Currents, swimming and danger of,
  8:98
Cushing's disease, 1:7
Cuspids (canines), 1:99
Cuticle (hair), 1:45
Cuticle (nail), 1:69
Cyanosis, 3:18

Cyclamate, 4:9
Cycling, 4:25–26
  on stationary bicycles, 4:40–41
  See also Fitness, 4:48–49; Fitness
    training, 4:49–50; Heart rate,
    4:68
Cyclones, 8:100
Cystic duct, 1:42
Cystic fibrosis, 1:23, 38, 77, 3:42–43.
  See also Lung, 1:62–63; Pancreas,
    1:76–77; Genetic screening,
    6:42–44; Genetic counselor, 9:12
Cystitis, 2:29, 3:80. *See also* Urinaly-
  sis, 1:100; Urinary tract,
    1:100–101; Bacterial infections,
    2:13–15; Inflammation, 2:51–52
Cysts, trichinosis and, 2:94, *94*
Cytoplasm, 1:23
Cytotechnologists, 9:23
Cytotoxic drugs. *See* Anticancer
  drugs

Dairy products. *See* Milk and milk
  products group
Dance, aerobic, 4:4
Dandruff, 3:43
Dandruff shampoo, 7:41. *See also* Pso-
  riasis, 3:98–99; Antifungal agents,
    7:24–25; Corticosteroids, 7:40
Darwin, Charles, 5:42
Date rape, 6:27–28. *See also* Violence,
    8:92–93
Dating, 6:28–29. *See also* Relationships, 5:82–83; Date rape, 6:27–28;
    Marriage, 6:55–56; Safer sex,
    6:82–83; Teenage pregnancy,
    6:97–98
DDI (dideoxyinosine), 2:7
DDT (dichlorodiphenyl-
  trichloroethane), 8:8, *48*, 92
Deafness, 1:34
  sensory, 8:59
  See also Hearing loss
Death, 1:28
  accidental, 8:5–6, *6*, 12, 13, 14,
    26, 51, 98
  autopsy after, 2:13
  caused by fire, 8:36
  dying and bereavement, 5:40–41
  from electric shock, 8:31
  by gunfire, 8:46
  by homicide, 8:53–54, 86, 92
  hospice care and, 9:18–19
  job-related, 8:79
  sudden cardiac, 3:71
  sudden infant death syndrome,
    3:108
  See also Violence, 8:92–93

Death syndrome, sudden infant, 3:108
Decibels, 8:59
Decline stage of infection, 2:50
Decompression chamber, 8:14
Decompression sickness. *See* Bends
Decongestants, 3:65, 7:25, 26–27, 52
  for common colds, 2:24
Deer tick, Lyme disease caused by,
    2:58
DEET, 7:68
Defecation, 1:10, 81
Defense mechanisms, 5:31–32. *See
  also* Anxiety, 5:9–10; Coping skills,
    5:29–30; Mind, 5:62–63; Self-
    efficacy, 5:88; Self-image, 5:89–90
Defensive driving, 8:13, 58
Defibrillator, 3:71
Defining attributes, 5:24
Deforestation
  carbon dioxide concentrations
    and, 8:21
  global warming and, 8:45–46
Degenerative joint disease. *See* Os-
  teoarthritis
Dehydration, 4:26–27, 124
  diarrhea and, 2:30
  drinking alcohol and, 7:61
  laxative overuse and, 7:70
  sports and heat problems caus-
    ing, 4:101–2
  sweating and, 4:26, 88, 101
  See also Beverages, 4:10–12
Delayed speaking, 3:104
Delirium tremens (DTs), 5:66, 7:42
  alcoholism and, 7:12–14
  hallucinations and, 5:48
  See also Addiction, 7:4–5; Alco-
    hol, 7:6–9; Drug rehabilitation,
    7:49–50; Withdrawal syn-
    drome, 7:100–101
Delta waves, 1:91
Deltoid muscles, 1:88
Delusions
  psychosis and, 5:78
  schizophrenia and, 5:86
Dementia, 3:9, 43–44
  AIDS, 2:6, 5:66
  senile, 5:90
  See also Syphilis, 2:87–88; Ane-
    mia, 3:11–12; Arteriosclerosis,
    3:15; Brain tumor, 3:25–26;
    Hypertension, 3:77–78; Stroke,
    3:106–8; Alcoholism, 7:12–14
Democratic leaders, 5:55
Dendrites, 1:74
Denial
  of alcoholism, 7:14
  of death, 5:40
  as defense mechanism, 5:31–32

Dental care, 9:7–8
  dental examination, 1:29
  toothpaste for, 7:99–100
  See also Tooth, 1:99–100; Dental
    problems, 3:44–45; Dentures,
    3:45–46; Gum disease,
    3:62–63; Orthodontic devices,
    3:92
Dental dams, 6:83
Dental examination, 1:29. *See also*
  Tooth, 1:99–100; Dental problems,
    3:44–45; Gum disease, 3:62–63;
    Dental care, 9:7–8
Dental hygienist, 1:29, 9:8
Dental problems, 3:44–45, *44*
  dentures, 3:45–46
  gum disease, 3:62–63
  orthodontic devices, 3:92
  See also Tooth, 1:99–100; Dental
    care, 9:7–8
Dentin, 1:99
Dentist, 3:44, 9:7
Dentures, 3:45–46. *See also* Dental
  care, 9:7–8
Deodorants, 7:42
Deoxyribonucleic acid (DNA), 1:22,
    4:117, 6:40, 63, 8:44
Department of Energy, 8:35
Department of Health and Human
  Services, 9:8–10. *See also* Food and
    Drug Administration, 7:59
Department of the Interior, 8:35
Dependence, drug, 5:40
  physical, 7:4–5, 8, 14, 73, 77, 88
  psychological, 7:4, 8, 73, 88
  steps to, 7:56–57
Dependent personality disorder,
    5:71
Depersonalization, 5:32
Depo-Provera, 6:26
Depressants, 7:6, 88
Depression, 5:32–34
  bipolar disorders and, 5:18–19,
    34
  over death, 5:40
  electroconvulsive therapy for,
    5:34, 41
  major, 5:33–34
  minor, 5:33
  postpartum, 6:73–74
  risk factors, 5:33
  suicide and, 5:33, 99, 100
  treatment of, 5:34, 7:23–24, 87
  See also Alienation, 5:6; Drug
    therapy, 5:39–40
Depression stage of dying, 5:40
Dermatitis, 2:76, 3:6, 43
  contact, 2:76, *76*, 3:6
  lice and, 2:57

Dermatologist, 1:90, 9:33
Dermis, 1:89, *90*
Desensitization, 5:17–18
Designated driver, 7:47
Designer drugs, 7:43. *See also* Amphetamines, 7:15; Drug use and abuse, 7:55–57; Narcotics, 7:76–78; Psychoactive drugs, 7:84–85
Despair, integrity versus, 5:36
Detached retina, 3:55, *55*
Detoxification, 7:14, 49–50
Developmental psychology, 5:34–36, 77
    environmental factors in, 5:50
    intellectual development, 5:34–35, 57
    moral development, 5:36
    social and emotional development, 5:35–36, 43
    See also Child development, 1:24–25; Heredity and environment, 5:49–50; Psychology, 5:76–78; Self-image, 5:89–90
Development stage of relationship, 5:83
Deviated septum, 1:76, 89
Diabetes, 1:9, 36, 65, 77, 3:10, 19, *20*, 46–48
    hyperglycemia and, 7:68
    insulin and, 7:68
    malnutrition and diabetes mellitus, 4:74
    See also Pancreas, 1:76–77
Diabetic diet, 4:32
Diagnostic and Statistical Manual of Mental Disorders (DSM), 5:60, 61, *61*
Dialysis, 3:48–49, *48. See also* Kidney, 1:57–58; Kidney disorders, 3:82–83
Diaper rash, 2:76
Diaphragm (contraceptive), 6:25, 29. *See also* Female reproductive system, 6:33–34; Fertilization, 6:35–37
Diaphragm (muscle), 1:30, *30*, 84
    hiccups and, 3:76–77
    See also Lung, 1:62–63; Respiratory system, 1:84–86
Diarrhea, 1:32, 2:29–30
    diverticulitis and, 3:49
    dysentery and, 2:31–32
    prevention and treatment of, 2:30, 7:24
    traveler's, 2:30, 4:58
Diastole, 1:48, *49*
Diastolic pressure, 1:15, 3:77
Dichlorodiphenyltrichloroethane (DDT), 8:8, *48*, 92
Dideoxyinosine (DDI), 2:7

Diet
    and aging, 1:9
    and blood diseases, 1:14
    and blood pressure, 1:15
    constipation and, 3:41, 75
    diabetes treatment and, 3:47
    and digestive problems, 1:33
    and endocrine system, 1:37
    and growth, 1:44
    and healthy bones, 1:18
    and heart disease, 1:49
    and kidney problems, 1:58
    and liver problems, 1:62
Diet aids, 4:27–28
    diet pills, 7:43–44
    diets and, 4:30–32
    diuretics and, 7:44–45
    exercise, 4:39–40
    fad diets, 4:42–43
    laxatives and, 7:69–70
    weight-loss strategy and, 4:128–30
    weight management and, 4:130–32
    See also Appetite, 4:8; Calorie(s), 4:20–21; Dietary guidelines, 4:28–29; Fiber, 4:47–48; Lifestyle, 4:71–72; Liposuction, 4:72; Nutrition, 4:84–85; Obesity, 4:85–86
Dietary guidelines, 4:28–29, *28*, 46
    for calories, 4:20–21
    for cholesterol, 4:23–24
    food group systems as, 4:55–56
    nutrients and, 4:82–84
    nutrition and, 4:84–85
    recommended dietary allowance (RDA) as, 4:92–93
    for weight management, 4:130–32
Dietetics, 4:85
Diet foods, 4:27, 29–30
    weight-loss strategy and, 4:128–30
    weight management and, 4:130–32
    See also Appetite, 4:8; Calorie(s), 4:20–21; Diet aids, 4:27–28; Dietary guidelines, 4:28–29; Diets, 4:30–32; Fats, 4:45–46; Food labeling, 4:56–57; Obesity, 4:85–86
Dietitians, 4:85, 9:26
Diet pills, 7:43–44
    appetite suppressants, 4:8, 27, 7:43–44, 95
    weight-loss strategy and, 4:128–30
    See also Diet aids, 4:27–28

Diets, 4:30–32
    carbohydrates in, 4:22
    controlling cholesterol with, 4:24
    dietary guidelines for, 4:28–29
    elements of healthy, 4:30
    exchange system for planning, 4:38–39
    fad, 4:42–43
    fiber in, 4:47–48
    food group systems and, 4:55–56
    food pyramid system to plan, 4:60–61
    macrobiotic, 4:73
    malnutrition caused by deficiencies in, 4:73–74
    nutrition and, 4:84–85
    risk factors in, 4:30, 95
    to treat and prevent illness, 4:31–32
    types of, 4:30–32, 42, 98–99
    vegetarian diet, 4:113–15
    water in, 4:123
    weight assessment and, 4:127
    for weight management, 4:131–32
    See also Appetite, 4:8; Diet foods, 4:29–30; Phytochemicals, 4:88–89
Diet success rate, 4:*129*
Diffusion of responsibility, 5:74
Digestion, 4:32–33, 54
    body metabolism and, 4:15–17
    See also Digestive system, 1:30–33; Appetite, 4:8; Energy, food, 4:35–36; Hunger, 4:68–69
Digestive enzymes, 1:31
Digestive system, 1:30–33, *31*
    gallbladder and, 1:42–43
    liver and, 1:60–62
    pancreas and, 1:76–77
    processes of, 4:32
    rectum and, 1:81
    salivary glands and, 1:86
    See also Diarrhea, 2:29–30; Gallstones, 3:58–59; Stomachache/indigestion, 3:105–6; Ulcer, peptic, 3:114–15; Dietary guidelines, 4:28–29
Dilation and curettage (D and C), 6:4, 5, 62
Dioxin, 8:92
Diphtheria, 2:30–31, *31*
    DPT vaccine for, 2:31, 90, 100
    See also Bacterial infections, 2:13–15; Immunization, 2:47–49

Direct-action anticoagulants, 7:23
Disabilities
    access for people with, 8:4–5
    learning, 5:58
Disability insurance, 9:16
Disaccharide, 4:110, 111
Discoid lupus erythematosus (DLE), 3:87
Discrimination, prejudice and, 5:73
Disease
    anger and, 5:7
    bacterial, 2:14, 15
    Centers for Disease Control and, 9:8–9, 9
    communicable, 2:24–26
    Legionnaires', 2:55–56
    Lyme, 2:58–59
    malnutrition caused by, 4:74
    stress and, 5:49, 97
Disinfectants, 7:29, 8:81
Disks, spinal, 1:94
Dislocations, 8:26, 26. See also Fractures, 8:41–43; Sprains and strains, 8:86–88
Displacement, 5:32
Dissolution of relationship, 5:83
Distillation, 7:6
Distress, 5:96
Disulfiram. See Antabuse
Diuretic(s), 3:78, 4:27, 7:44–45, 53
    alcohol as, 7:61
    as antihypertensives, 7:27, 44
    in diet pills, 7:43, 44
    See also Laxatives, 7:69–70
Divergent thinking, 5:30
Diverticulitis, 3:49. See also Digestive system, 1:30–33; Diarrhea, 2:29–30; Fiber, 4:47–48
Diverticulosis, 2:30, 3:49
Diving safety, underwater, 8:99
Divorce, 5:36–37. See also Family, 5:44–45; Love, 5:58–59; Relationships, 5:82–83; Marriage, 6:55–56; Spouse abuse, 8:86
D-limonene, 4:89
DMSO, 9:38
DNA (deoxyribonucleic acid), 1:22, 4:117, 6:40, 8:44
    mutation and altered, 6:63
Doctor, when to call a, 8:57
Doctors of Osteopathy (D.O.'s). See Osteopathic physicians (D.O.'s)
Doctors of Medicine (M.D.'s). See Physicians (M.D.'s)
Domestic violence, 8:92, 93
Dominant genes, 6:41
Dominant inheritance, 6:41
Donor cards for transplants, 3:113
Dopamine, 3:95, 96, 96, 7:70

Dosage, 7:45–46
    drug overdose, 7:48–49
    See also Body metabolism, 4:15–17; Drug use and abuse, 7:55–57
Dose-response relationship, 7:45
Double-blind, crossover trials, 7:37
Double-blind food allergy test, 3:9
Double-blind studies, 7:37
Douching, 6:35
Down syndrome, 1:23, 3:49–50, 50, 6:11, 42. See also Genetic screening, 6:42–44; Genetic counselor, 9:12
DPT (diphtheria, pertussis, tetanus) vaccine, 2:31, 90, 100
Dreams, 5:37–39
    effects of, on body, 5:38, 38
    nature of, 5:38
    nocturnal emissions and, 6:67
    significance of, 5:38–39
    sleep and, 1:92
    See also Sleep disorders, 3:103–4; Psychiatry, 5:75; Sleep problems, 5:93–94
Drinking and driving, 7:8, 9, 46–47, 8:12. See also Alcohol, 7:6–9; Alcoholism, 7:12–14; Intoxication, 7:68–69; Social drinking, 7:92–93
Drives, 5:64
Driving. See Automobile safety; Drinking and driving; Motorcycle safety
Drought, emergencies caused by, 8:99–100
Drowning, 8:26–27
    water safety to prevent, 8:27, 98–99
    See also CPR, 8:24–25; Hypothermia, 8:54–55
Drug allergy, 3:6, 7:47. See also Allergies, 3:6–8; Shock, 3:101; Drugs, 7:50–52
Drug approval process, 7:37, 37
Drug interaction, 7:47–48
    alcohol and, 7:23, 26, 48
    antibiotics and, 7:23, 48
    anticoagulant use and, 7:23
    antidepressants and, 7:24
    antihistamines and, 7:26, 48
    aspirin and, 7:23, 30
    blocked effect, 7:48
    caffeine and, 7:35
    dosage and, 7:45–46
    heroin and, 7:63
    increased effects, 7:48
    L-dopa and, 7:70
    marijuana and, 7:72
    methadone and, 7:74
    preventing harmful, 7:48

    sedatives and, 7:88
    sleeping pills and, 7:90
Drug overdose, 7:48–49, 63. See also Drug use and abuse, 7:55–57
Drug profile, 9:30
Drug rehabilitation, 7:5, 49–50
    course of treatment, 7:49–50
    for heroin addiction, 7:5, 16, 49–50, 63, 74
    methadone used in, 7:16, 50, 74
    post-treatment support, 7:50
    recovery, 7:50
    See also Alcoholism, 7:12–14; Codependency, 7:39–40; Drug use and abuse, 7:55–57
Drugs, 7:50–52
    AIDS and intravenous (IV) drug use, 2:4
    anesthetic, 7:17
    anticancer, 7:22–23
    anticoagulants, 7:23
    antidepressants, 7:23–24
    antihistamines and decongestants, 7:25–27
    antihypertensive, 7:27
    anti-inflammatory, 7:28
    antipsychotic, 5:39, 39, 40, 81, 86
    antiviral, 7:29–30
    anxiolytics, 7:87, 90
    clinical drug trials, 7:37
    designer, 7:43
    dosage of, 7:45–46
    driving and use of, 8:12
    generic, 7:52, 59–60
    hallucinogens, 5:48
    immunosuppressants, 7:65
    look-alike, 7:70
    medicinal, 7:51–52
    methods of classifying, 7:50–51, 51
    nonprescription, 7:78–79
    opportunistic infections and, 2:68
    organic brain disorders and, 5:66
    poisoning by, 8:67–68
    psychoactive, 7:51, 52, 84–85
    recreational, 7:6, 52
    sulfa, 7:96–97
    vasodilator, 3:19, 78, 7:27
    violence and abuse of, 8:92
    See also Addiction, 7:4–5; Drugs and the law, 7:53–54; Drug use and abuse, 7:55–57
Drugs and sports, 7:52–53. See also Drug use and abuse, 7:55–57
Drugs and the law, 7:53–54, 55. See also Drug rehabilitation, 7:49–50; Drug use and abuse, 7:55–57

Drug testing, 7:52, 54–55, 94
  blood alcohol level (BAL), 7:33–34
  in sports, 7:52–53
  See also Drug use and abuse, 7:55–57
Drug therapy, 5:39–40, *39*, 81
  antidepressants for, 7:23–24
  benefits and costs of, 5:39–40
  for bipolar disorder, 5:19
  for depression, 5:34
  for hyperactivity, 5:51
  for mental illness, 5:61
  sedatives for, 7:87–88
  types of, 5:39, *39*
  See also Addiction, 7:4–5; Tolerance, 7:99
Drug use and abuse, 7:55–57
  administering drugs, 7:56
  agent-host-environment model of, 7:57
  alcoholism, 7:12–14
  drug testing for, 7:54–55
  during pregnancy, 6:12
  steps to drug dependency, 7:56–57
  See also Drug interaction, 7:47–48; Psychoactive drugs, 7:84–85
Dry gangrene, 3:59, *59*
Drying, food preservation by, 4:59
Dry pleurisy, 3:98
DTs. *See* Delirium tremens (DTs)
Duchenne muscular dystrophy, 3:90, 91
Duodenal ulcers, 3:114, *115*
Duodenum, 1:32
Dwarfism, 3:61
Dwarf tapeworms, 2:89
Dying and bereavement, 5:40–41
  hospice program and, 9:18–19
  See also Death, 1:28
Dyscalcula, 5:58
Dysentery, 2:31–32
  amebic, 2:31, 69
  See also Diarrhea, 2:29–30
Dysfunctional families, 5:45
Dysgraphia, 5:58
Dyskinetic cerebral palsy, 3:37
Dyslexia, 5:21, 58
Dysmenorrhea, 6:60
Dyspepsia. *See* Indigestion (dyspepsia)
Dysphasia, 5:58
Dysplasia, cervical, 6:69

Ear, 1:33–34, *33. See also* Hearing loss, 3:66–67

Earaches, 1:34
Eardrops, 7:57–58. *See also* Ear infections, 2:32–34; Antibiotics, 7:20–22; Corticosteroids, 7:40
Eardrum, 1:34, 3:67
Ear infections, 2:32–34, *33*
  eardrops for, 7:57
  hearing loss and, 3:67
Early adulthood, 1:8
  gender identity in, 6:40
Early school stage, 1:25
Earthquakes, 8:27–29
  areas prone to, 8:28, *28*
  preparedness for, 8:28–29
  See also Weather-related emergencies, 8:99–101
Earwax, buildup of, 3:67
Eating disorders, 4:8, 33–34, 74
  anorexia/bulimia, 5:8
  food craving, 4:54–55
  malnutrition, 4:73–75
  psychological characteristics of people with, 5:8
  See also Fasting, 4:43–44; Underweight, 4:113; Weight assessment, 4:124–27
Echocardiogram, 3:72, 73
Ecosystem, 8:29, *29*
  agricultural pollution and, 8:8
  in biosphere, 8:15
  See also Acid rain, 8:6–7; Thermal pollution, 8:91
Ecstasy, 7:43
Ectopic pregnancy, 2:70, 6:10, 36–37, 52, 75
Eczema, 2:33, 76, 3:6, 51. *See also* Antihistamines and decongestants, 7:25–27; Corticosteroids, 7:40
Edema, 1:64, 98, 4:124
  diuretics to treat, 7:44
Educator, health, 9:15–16
Effective dose, 7:45
Effluent, 8:82, 91
Egg cells (ova), 1:83
Eggs, *Salmonella* contamination of, 4:62
Eighteenth Amendment to Constitution, 7:53
Ejaculation, 1:83, 6:54, 91, 93
  nocturnal emission, 6:54, 67, 80
  orgasm and, 6:67
  premature, 6:88–89
  semen discharged by, 6:84
Elastic cartilage, 1:27
Elbow, 1:34–35, *35*
  See also Connective tissue, 1:27–28; Joint, 1:56; Musculoskeletal system, 1:68–69; Tendinitis, 3:111–12

Elderly
  malnutrition among, 4:75
  suicide among, 5:100
Electrical injuries, 8:52
Electrical safety, 8:30–31
  accidents and, 8:6, 30, 52
  in home, 8:30–31, 52, 78
  See also Burns, 8:20–21; Electric shock, 8:31; Fire safety, 8:36–37
Electric blankets, 8:30
Electric conductivity, 4:14, 127
Electricity, nuclear power for, 8:61–62
Electric shock, 3:101, 8:31, *31*
Electrocardiogram (ECG or EKG), 3:51–52, 72
  stress test, 3:52, 106
  See also Heart, 1:47–49; Heart attack, 3:68–69
Electroconvulsive therapy (ECT), 5:41, 81
  for depression, 5:34, 41
  See also Drug therapy, 5:39–40
Electroencephalogram (EEG), 2:34, 3:52, 54, *54*
Electromagnetic radiation, 8:73
Elevation of injured area, 8:77
ELISA test, 2:6
Embolism, 3:14, 19, 24, 86
Embolus, 3:14, *24*
Embryo, 6:30–31, *31*, 36, 37, 40. *See also* Female reproductive system, 6:33–34; Fertilization, 6:35–37; Fetus, 6:37–38; Pregnancy, 6:74–76
Emergencies, weather-related. *See* Weather-related emergencies
Emergency care center, 8:33
Emergency care services, 8:32–33, 38. *See also* First aid, 8:38–39; Poison-Control Centers, 8:66–67; Emergency medical technician, 9:10–11; Hospital, 9:19–20
Emergency department, 9:20
Emergency first aid, 8:38–39, *38, 39*
Emergency medical identification, 8:33
Emergency medical technician (EMT), 8:32, 9:10–11
  EMT-ambulance, 9:10
  EMT-intermediate, 9:10
  EMT-paramedic, 9:10–11
Emergency Medicine Specialists, 9:33
Emergency procedures. *See* First aid
Emotion, 5:42–44
  anger, 5:7–8
  anxiety, 5:9–10
  depression, 5:32–34
  fear, 5:45–46

happiness, 5:48–49
love, 5:58–59
theories of, 5:42–43, 43
See also Immune system, 1:52–55; Psychosomatic disorders, 5:78–79
Emotional abuse of children, 8:23
Emotional aspect of communication, 5:23
Emotional changes in puberty, 6:80
Emotional costs of divorce, 5:37
Emotional development, 5:35–36, 43
Emotional health, 5:60
Emotional intimacy, 5:54
Empathy, 5:23
Emphysema, 1:63, 85, 2:17, 18, 3:18, 53, 53, 7:91. See also Lung, 1:62–63; Bronchitis, 2:17–18; Smoking, 7:90–92
Empty calories, 4:70, 97
Emulsifiers, 4:53
Enamel, tooth, 1:99
Encephalitis, 2:34
organic brain disorders and, 5:66
palsy and, 3:37
Endemic typhus, 2:96
Endocarditis, 2:34–35, 35, 3:71, 73. See also Heart, 1:47–49; Bacterial infections, 2:13–15; Heart disease, 3:69–72
Endocardium, 1:47, 2:34
Endocrine glands, 1:43
Endocrine system, 1:35–37, 36
adrenal glands, 1:6–7
general adaptation syndrome and, 5:96
pituitary gland, 1:79–80
sex hormones produced by, 6:84–85
thyroid gland, 1:96–97
See also Nervous system, 1:71–74; Thyroid disorders, 3:112
Endometriosis, 6:31–32
hysterectomy due to, 6:32, 48
infertility caused by, 6:51
See also Female reproductive system, 6:33–34; Pregnancy, 6:74–76
Endometritis, 2:70
Endometrium, 6:36, 59, 60
Endorphins, 1:37
acupuncture and release of, 3:5, 7:87
placebos and release of, 7:82
See also Pituitary gland, 1:79–80; Pain, 3:94
Endoscope, 3:114
Endoscopic biopsy, 3:22–23

End-stage renal failure, 3:83
Endurance, 4:34–35, 49
aerobic exercise for, 4:35, 50
cardiovascular, 4:34, 35, 49
muscular, 4:34, 35, 49, 99, 100
See also Exercise, 4:39–40; Fitness, 4:48–49; Strength exercise, 4:108–9; Weight training, 4:132–33
Enema, barium, 3:39
Energy
conservation, 8:33–34, 34
Department of Energy and, 8:35
nuclear, 8:61–62
recycling to save, 8:75
solar, 8:83–84
Energy, food, 4:14–15, 35–36
calories and, 4:20–21
sugar as, 4:110–11
See also Body metabolism, 4:15–17; Energy, physical, 4:36–38; Nutrients, 4:82–84; Weight management, 4:130–32
Energy, physical, 4:36–38, 37
exercise and, 4:39–40
See also Energy, food, 4:35–36; Nutrients, 4:82–84; Rest, 4:93–94; Weight management, 4:130–32
Energy-balance equation, 4:20–21, 36, 131
Energy conservation, 8:33–34, 34, 40–41, 41
solar energy and, 8:83–84
Enriched breads, 4:17
Environment
exposure to radiation in, 8:73
population growth and, 8:71
recycling and protection of, 8:74–76
unsafe, accidents due to, 8:6
See also Heredity and environment, 5:49–50
Environmental carcinogens, 3:33
Environmental factors in agent-host-environment model, 7:57
Environmental organizations, 8:35, 90. See also Ecosystem, 8:29; Global warming, 8:45–46; Ozone, 8:64–65
Environmental Protection Agency (EPA), 7:92, 8:8, 35, 65, 74, 76
Superfund, 8:49, 89–90
Environmental psychology, 5:77–78
Enzyme, 1:31, 32, 37–38, 76
food spoilage and, 4:59
muscular endurance and, 4:35
pancreatic, 1:32, 76
See also Cystic fibrosis, 3:42–43

Epicanthic folds, fetal alcohol syndrome and, 7:58
Epicardium, 1:47
Epidemic, 2:36
AIDS, 2:5
cholera, 2:22–23
influenza, 2:52–53
plague, 2:71–72
See also Antibiotic treatment, 2:8–10; Communicable diseases, 2:24–26; Epidemiology, 2:36–37; Immunization, 2:47–49; Microorganisms, 2:63–65; Poliomyelitis, 2:73–74
Epidemic typhus, 2:96
Epidemiologists, 2:36
Epidemiology, 2:36–37. See also Epidemic, 2:36
Epidermis, 1:89
Epididymis, 6:53
Epiglottis, 1:32, 95
Epilepsy, 3:53–54. See also Nervous system, 1:71–74; Neuron, 1:74–75; Stroke, 3:106–8; Body metabolism, 4:15–17
Epinephrine, 1:7, 36, 38–39, 51, 52, 3:8
for anaphylactic shock, 7:47
basal metabolic rate and, 4:16
nicotine and stimulation of, 7:98
See also Hormone(s), 1:51–52; Stress, 5:95–98; Stress-management techniques, 5:98–99
Epiphysis, 1:18
Episiotomy, 6:20
Epithelial tissue, 1:98
Epstein-Barr virus, 3:38
mononucleosis caused by, 2:65
Equipment
safety, 8:77–79
self-care, 8:57
unsafe, accidents due to, 8:5–6
Erection, 6:54
Ergometers, 4:41
Erikson, Erik, 5:35–36
Erotica, 6:90
Erythrocytes. See Red blood cells (erythrocytes)
Erythromycin, 2:87
Escherichia coli (E. coli), 2:13, 14
diarrhea from, 4:58
Esophagus, 1:31, 31, 32, 70, 70, 95, 95, 96
Essential amino acids, 4:76, 90
Essential hypertension, 3:78
Estrogen, 1:7, 18
atrophic vaginitis and deficiency of, 6:102

in birth-control pill, 6:9
function of, 6:85
hormone therapy with, 7:63, 64
ovulation and, 6:68
produced by placenta, 6:72
puberty and, 6:79
Estrogen replacement therapy (ERT), 1:18, 3:93, 6:58
Ethanol. See Alcohol
Ethics
    of genetic engineering, 8:45
    medical, 9:21–22
    use of placebos and, 7:82
Ethmoid sinuses, 1:88
Ethyl alcohol. See Alcohol
Eustachian tube, 1:5, 34
    middle-ear infections and, 2:33
Eustress, 5:95–96
Euthanasia, 9:21
Eutrophication, 8:96
Examination
    breast self-examination, 6:15–17, 16
    dental, 1:29
    gynecological, 6:44–45
    physical, 1:78–79
    testicular self-examination, 6:98–99
Exchange system, 4:38–39. See also Dietary guidelines, 4:28–29; Five food groups system, 4:50–51; Food group systems, 4:55–56; Food pyramid system, 4:60–61; Four food groups system, 4:64–65
Excretory system, 1:39
    kidney and, 1:57–58
    liver and, 1:60–62
    perspiration and, 4:87–88
    urinary tract and, 1:100–101
    See also Digestive system, 1:30–33; Lung, 1:62–63; Respiratory system, 1:84–86
Exercise, 4:39–40
    aerobic, 4:4–6
    aerobic dance for, 4:4
    and aging, 1:9
    anaerobic, 4:7
    asthma and, 3:19
    body composition and, 4:13
    and bones, 1:18
    calories and energy expenditure in, 4:20–21
    cross training, 4:24–25
    diabetes treatment and, 3:47
    and endocrine system, 1:37
    fitness and, 4:48
    fitness training and, 4:49–50
    forms of, 4:39–40
    and good night's sleep, 1:92

health and, 4:39
in hot weather, 8:49, 50
lifestyle and, 4:40
metabolic rate and, 4:16, 17
and musculoskeletal disorders, 1:69
osteoporosis prevention and, 3:93
physical therapists' use of, 9:31
precautions about, 4:40
relaxation after, 4:93
risk factors based on, 4:95
strength, 4:108–9
stress management with, 5:29, 98
sweating and fluid replacement during, 4:88, 101, 102
to treat obesity, 4:86
walking for, 4:122–23
weight-loss strategy and, 4:129
weight management and, 4:132
See also Energy, physical, 4:36–38; Exercise machines, 4:40–42; Risk factors, 4:94–95; Sports and fitness, 4:99–101; Sports and heat problems, 4:101–2; Sports injuries, 4:102–5; Sports medicine, 4:105–6
Exercise machines, 4:40–42, 132
    weight training with, 4:132–33
    See also Cross training, 4:24–25; Endurance, 4:34–35; Fitness training, 4:49–50
Exercise tolerance test. See Stress test
Exhaustion stage of general adaptation syndrome, 5:96
Exhibitionism, 6:9
Exocrine glands, 1:43
Expectation, perception and, 5:68, 68
Expectorants, 2:17, 7:41
Experimental psychology, 5:77
Experimentation in adolescence, 1:6
Extended family, 5:44, 45
External bleeding, 8:18
Exxon Valdez (oil tanker), 8:63–64
Eye, 1:39–41, 40
    Chlamydia trachomatis infection of, 2:21
    conjunctivitis of, 2:26–27
    fluid drainage in, 3:60, 60
    poisonous substances in, 8:69
    yellow whites of, jaundice and, 3:81
    See also Eye disorders, 3:54–55; Eye care, 9:11–12
Eye care, 9:11–12
    eye test, 3:55
    vision problems and, 3:116–17
    See also Eye disorders, 3:54–55

Eye disorders, 3:54–55, 83
    cataracts, 3:35–36, 35
    eye care and, 9:11–12
    eye tests for, 3:55
    glaucoma, 3:60
    See also Eye, 1:39–41; Thyroid disorders, 3:112; Vision problems, 3:116–17
Eyedrops, 7:58
    for conjunctivitis, 2:26–27
    See also Antibiotics, 7:20–22; Antihistamines and decongestants, 7:25–27; Corticosteroids, 7:40
Eyeglasses, 3:117
Eye tests, 3:54, 55, 60. See also Vision problems, 3:116–17; Eye care, 9:11–12
Eyewashes, 7:58

Face lifts, 3:97
Facial bones, 1:91
Facial expression of anger, 5:7
Fad diets, 4:42–43, 130
    quackery involved in, 9:38
    See also Diet aids, 4:27–28; Diets, 4:30–32; Fasting, 4:43–44; Malnutrition, 4:73–75; Obesity, 4:85–86; Weight management, 4:130–32
Failure to thrive, 8:23
Fainting, 3:55–56
Fallopian tubes, 1:83, 6:33
    ectopic pregnancy in, 2:70
    fertilization in, 6:35–36, 36
    tubal ligation, 6:25, 96, 96
Falls, 8:5, 51–52
Familial polyposis, 1:81
Family, 5:44–45
    challenges for, 5:44–45
    child abuse in, 8:22–23
    divorce and, 5:36–37
    happiness and, 5:48
    importance of, 5:45
    incest within, 6:49–50
    marriage and, 6:55–56
    parenthood and, 6:69–71
    relationships within, 5:82–83
    sibling rivalry in, 5:92
    spouse abuse in, 8:86
    types of, 5:44
Family adoptions, 6:6
Family planning, 8:71
    contraception and, 6:24–26
    natural, 6:5, 24, 25, 66
Family practitioners, 9:32
Family therapy, 5:81
Fantasies, sexual, 6:89–90

Farsightedness, 3:*116*, 117
Fast food, 4:43. *See also* Fats, oils, and sweets group, 4:46–47; Junk food, 4:70–71
Fasting, 4:43–44. *See also* Fad diets, 4:42–43; Weight-loss strategy, 4:128–30
Fat, body. *See* Body fat
Fat cells, 1:90, 4:15, 72
Fatfold measurement, 4:14, 126
Fatigue, 4:44–45
    chronic fatigue syndrome and, 3:38
    See also Sleep, 1:91–92; Anemia, 3:11–12; Malnutrition, 4:73–75
Fats, 4:45–46, *46, 83, 83*
    in fast foods, 4:43
    low-fat diet, 4:31
    in meat, eggs, and legumes group, 4:77
    saturated, 4:24, *24,* 45, 46, 47, 77
    unsaturated, 4:45–46
    vegetarian diet and, 4:115
    weight-gain strategy and, 4:128
    See also Body fat, 4:14–15; Carbohydrates, 4:21–22; Energy, food, 4:35–36; Fats, oils, and sweets group, 4:46–47; Nutrients, 4:82–84; Obesity, 4:85–86; Proteins, 4:90–92
Fats, oils, and sweets group, 4:46–47, 51, 60. *See also* Atherosclerosis, 3:19–20; Breast cancer, 3:26–28; Colorectal cancer, 3:40; Heart disease, 3:69–72; Dietary guidelines, 4:28–29; Exchange system, 4:38–39; Food group systems, 4:55–56
Fat-soluble vitamins, 4:118, 119, 120, *121,* 122
Fatty acids, 4:14, 36
FDA. *See* Food and Drug Administration (FDA)
Fear, 5:45–46
    anxiety compared to, 5:10
    desensitization to overcome, 5:17–18
    See also Anxiety disorders, 5:10–12; Stress, 5:95–98
Fearlessness, 5:46
Fecal impaction, 3:80
Fecal incontinence, 3:80
Feces, 1:10, 32, 81
    bowel movements and, 3:41–42
    diarrhea and, 2:29–30
    laxative and removal of, 7:69–70
Federal Trade Commission (FTC), 9:38

Feedback, 5:22, 57. *See also* Biofeedback, 5:18
Feingold, Benjamin, 5:51
Fellatio, 6:67
Female pattern baldness, 3:63
Female reproductive system, 1:83–84, *83,* 6:33–34, *34*
    childbirth and, 6:20–21
    gynecological examination of, 6:44–45
    menopause and, 6:58–59
    menstrual cycle, 6:59–60, *59,* 85
    See also Breast self-examination, 6:15–17; Feminine hygiene, 6:34–35; Male reproductive system, 6:52–54
Female sex hormones, 6:85
Female sexual dysfunction, 6:89
Feminine hygiene, 6:34–35, 60. *See also* Toxic shock syndrome (TSS), 2:92–93
Femoral hernia, 3:76
Femur, 1:50, 58
Fermentation, 7:6
Fertility testing, 6:51
Fertilization, 6:30, 33, 35–37, *36*
    cell division, 6:36, 40
    contraception and, 6:24–26
    ectopic pregnancy and, 2:70, 6:10, 36–37, 52, 75
    implantation, 6:36
    infertility and, 6:50–51
    ovulation and, 6:68
    pregnancy and, 6:74–76
    sexual intercourse and, 6:91–92
    See also Female reproductive system, 6:33–34; Genetics, 6:40–42; Male reproductive system, 6:52–54; Menstruation, 6:59–61
Fertilizers, 4:6, 86, 8:7, 8
Fetal alcohol syndrome (FAS), 6:12, 38, 78, 7:58–59. *See also* Birth defects, 6:11–12; Fetus, 6:37–38
Fetal distress, 6:19
Fetishism, 6:9
Fetus, 1:83, 6:30, 36, 37–38, *38,* 74–75
    amniotic fluid surrounding, 6:7, *7,* 20
    birth defects in, 6:11–12
    placenta and, 6:71–72
    ultrasound to view, 6:100
    umbilical cord and, 6:101, *101*
    See also Fetal alcohol syndrome, 7:58–59
Fever, 1:53, 2:37–38
    paratyphoid, 2:96
    rheumatic, 2:77–78

    scarlet, 2:81–82
    typhoid, 2:96
    when to call doctor about, 8:57
    See also Infection, 2:50–51; Reye's syndrome, 3:100
Fever blister. *See* Cold sore
FSH (follicle-stimulating hormone), 1:*51,* 80, *80,* 6:84
Fiber, 3:32, 40, 41, 4:21, 47–48, *48*
    low- and high-fiber diets, 4:31–32
    vegetarian diet and, 4:115
    See also Carbohydrates, 4:21–22; Dietary guidelines, 4:28–29
Fibrocartilage, 1:27
Fibroids, 6:48, 51
Fibrositis, 3:56. *See also* Sleep disorders, 3:103–4
Fibula, 1:10
Fight-or-flight response, 1:7, 38–39, 5:10, 16, 42
Fingers, 1:23, 46
    Raynaud's phenomenon and, 3:100
Finger sweep, 8:24
Firearms. *See* Gun control
Fire drills, 8:37
Fire extinguisher, 8:36, 37, 52, 77
Fire safety, 8:36–37
    electrical accidents and, 8:30
    in home, 8:52–53, 77
    smoke inhalation, preventing, 8:83
    tips for, 8:37
    See also Burns, 8:20–21; Home safety, 8:51–53
First aid, 8:38–39
    for burns, 8:20–21
    CPR as, 8:24–25, *25,* 31, 38
    for drowning, 8:27
    for electric shock, 8:31, *31*
    emergency, 8:38–39, *38, 39*
    for external bleeding, 8:18
    for fractures, 8:42
    for frostbite, 8:43
    Heimlich maneuver, 8:50–51
    for internal bleeding, 8:19
    for minor injuries, 8:38
    for poisoning, 8:68–69
    RICE technique, 8:76–77, *76,* 87
    for smoke inhalation, 8:83
    for sprains and strains, 8:55–56, 87
    for wounds, 8:18, 101
    See also Medicine cabinet, 7:73–74; Accidents, 8:5–6; Emergency medical technician, 9:10–11
First aid kit, 8:38, 39–40

First Amendment of the Constitution, 6:73
First-degree burns, 8:20, *20*
Fish, 4:75–76
Fission, nuclear, 8:61, 62
Fitness, 4:48–49
    aerobic exercise and, 4:4–6
    body metabolism and, 4:17
    cardiovascular, 4:4, 5, 6, 68, 100
    President's Council on Physical
      Fitness and Sports, 4:90
    running for, 4:95–96
    sports and, 4:99–101
    swimming for, 4:112
    walking for, 4:122–23
    See also Body composition,
      4:13–14; Endurance, 4:34–35;
      Flexibility, 4:51–52; Strength,
      4:107; Weight assessment,
      4:124–27
Fitness training, 4:49–50
    cross training and, 4:24–25
    See also Energy, physical,
      4:36–38; Sports and fitness,
      4:99–101
Five food groups system, 4:50–51.
    See also Dietary guidelines,
      4:28–29; Exchange system,
      4:38–39; Food group systems,
      4:55–56; Food pyramid system,
      4:60–61; Four food groups system,
      4:64–65
Fixed braces, 3:92
Flammable materials, storing, 8:36
Flashbacks, hallucinogenic, 7:61, 71
Flat breads, 4:17
Flat feet, 3:57
Flatulence, 3:105
Flavoring agents, 4:52
    artificial sweeteners, 4:8–9
    monosodium glutamate (MSG),
      4:82
Fleas, 2:71, 96
Fleming, Alexander, 7:20, 80
Flexibility, 4:13, 49, 51–52
    stretching exercise for, 4:50,
      51–52
    See also Fitness training,
      4:49–50; Sports injuries,
      4:102–5; Strength exercise,
      4:108–9
Floods, 8:100
Flossing, 1:99, 3:45, 63
Flu. *See* Influenza
Flukes (parasitic worms), 2:64
Fluorescent light bulbs, 8:34
Fluoride, 4:*80*, 81, 7:99–100
Flu shots, 2:53
Fogarty International Center, 9:9

Folic acid, 4:*116*, 117, *121*
Folic acid anemia, 3:12
Folk medicine, 4:89
    hallucinogens in, 7:61
Follicles, 1:45
    hair, 3:4, *4*
Follicle-stimulating hormone (FSH),
    1:*51*, 80, *80*, 6:84
Food(s)
    allergies to certain, 3:6, 7
    cancer and, 3:32
    contamination of, 4:62–63
    diet, 4:27, 29–30
    genetically engineered, 8:44
    migraine triggered by, 3:89
    organic, 4:86, 8:8
    stomachache/indigestion due to,
      3:105–6
Food additives, 4:52–53, 63
    food preservation methods and,
      4:59–60
    See also Food allergies, 4:53–54;
      Food labeling, 4:56–57; Food
      safety, 4:61–63; Organic food,
      4:86; Food and Drug Adminis-
      tration (FDA), 7:59
Food allergies, 4:53–54. *See also* Al-
    lergies, 3:6–8
Food allergy test, double-blind, 3:9
Food and Drug Administration
    (FDA), 1:14, 3:97, 4:8, 27, 29, 47,
    52, 53, 57, 6:15, 24, 7:59, 8:44,
    9:8, 38
    AZT, approval of, 7:31
    bioequivalence requirements of
      generic drugs, 7:59, 60
    diet pills, approval of, 7:44
    drug approval process, 7:37, *37*
    nonprescription drug regulation
      by, 7:78
Food and Nutrition Board of National
    Academy of Sciences, 4:56
Food chain, toxic chemicals in, 8:96
Food craving, 4:54–55, *55*. *See also*
    Appetite, 4:8; Weight management,
    4:130–32
Food, Drug and Cosmetic Act
    (1962), 7:78
Food energy. *See* Energy, food
Food group systems, 4:55–56
    breads and cereals group,
      4:17–18
    exchange system, 4:38–39
    fats, oils, and sweets group,
      4:46–47
    five food groups system, 4:50–51
    food pyramid system, 4:60–61
    four food groups system,
      4:64–65, *64*

    fruits and vegetables group,
      4:65–66
    meats, eggs, and legumes group,
      4:75–77
    milk and milk products group,
      4:77–78
    See also Dietary guidelines,
      4:28–29
Food intolerance, 4:54
Food labeling, 4:56–57
    for diet foods, 4:29
    for organic foods, 4:86
    RDAs and, 4:56, 93
    for snack foods, 4:97
    for sodium, 4:99
    See also Dietary guidelines,
      4:28–29; Food and Drug Ad-
      ministration, 7:59
Food poisoning, 4:57–58, 62, 63
    botulism, 2:14
    salmonella, 2:80, 4:57, 62
    See also Bacterial infections,
      2:13–15; Diarrhea, 2:29–30;
      Parasitic infections, 2:68–69;
      Salmonella infections, 2:80;
      Trichinosis, 2:94; Viral infec-
      tions, 2:97–98; Vomiting,
      2:98–99; Food safety, 4:61–63
Food preservation methods, 4:52,
    59–60. *See also* Food safety,
    4:61–63; Food and Drug Adminis-
    tration, 7:59
Food product dating, 4:57
Food pyramid system, 4:60–61, *61*.
    See also Dietary guidelines, 4:28–29;
    Exchange system, 4:38–39; Five
    food groups system, 4:50–51; Food
    group systems, 4:55–56; Four food
    groups system, 4:64–65; Nutrients,
    4:82–84
Food safety, 4:58, 61–63, 8:81
    food allergies and, 4:53–54
    food labeling and, 4:56–57
    See also Bacterial infections,
      2:13–15; Salmonella infections,
      2:80
Food spoilage, 4:59
Foot, 1:41–42, *41*
    arches of, 1:42, 3:57
    See also Podiatrist, 9:34
Foot problems, 3:57–58
    athlete's foot, 2:12
    blisters, 3:23–24
    podiatrist for, 9:34
    sports and, 4:103, *103*
    See also Podiatrist, 9:34
Foreskin of penis, circumcision of,
    6:21–22, *22*, 54
Forest Service, 8:35

Formal operational stage, 5:35
Fortified cereals, 4:17
Fossil fuels, use of, 8:40–41
    acid rain from, 8:6–7, 7, 40
    air pollution and, 8:9–10, 40
    carbon dioxide produced in, 8:21
    conservation in, 8:33, 40–41
    greenhouse effect and, 8:45, 45
    industrial smog from, 8:82
    oil spills, 8:63–64
Foster parents, 6:70
Four food groups system, 4:64–65,
    64. See also Dietary guidelines,
    4:28–29; Exchange system,
    4:38–39; Five food groups system,
    4:50–51; Food group systems,
    4:55–56; Food pyramid system,
    4:60–61
Fourth Amendment to Constitution,
    7:55
Fovea, 1:40
Fracture, bone, 3:93, 118, 8:41–43,
    42
    first aid for, 8:42
    medical treatment for, 8:42
    recovery process, 8:42–43
    types of, 8:41, 42
    See also Osteoporosis, 3:93; X-ray
        examination, 3:117–18; Acci-
        dents, 8:5–6; Dislocations,
        8:26
Fraternal siblings, 6:62–63, 62
Free association, 5:79
Freebasing, 7:38
Free-floating anxiety, 5:10
Free radicals, 4:10, 89, 117, 119
Free weights, 4:42, 132
Freeze-drying, 4:59
Freezing method of preserving foods,
    4:59
Freud, Sigmund, 5:31, 38, 43, 63, 75,
    76, 79, 9:36
Friendship, 5:46–47, 83
    happiness and, 5:48
    health and, 5:47
    See also Communication,
        5:22–23; Intimacy, 5:54; Love,
        5:58–59; Relationships,
        5:82–83; Responsibility,
        5:84–85; Social skills, 5:94–95
Frontal lobe, 1:21, 5:21
Frontal sinuses, 1:88
Frostbite, 8:43, 101. See also Gan-
    grene, 3:59; Hypothermia, 8:54–55
Fructose, 4:111
Fruit drinks, 4:11–12
Fruits and vegetables group,
    4:50–51, 60, 64, 64, 65–66. See
    also Dietary guidelines, 4:28–29;

Exchange system, 4:38–39; Five
food groups system, 4:50–51; Food
pyramid system, 4:60–61; Four
food groups system, 4:64–65
Functional disorders, 5:61
Fungal infections, 2:38–39
    athlete's foot, 2:12
    candida infections, 2:19
    in nails, 1:69
    treatment and prevention of,
        2:39, 7:24–25
    types of, 2:39
    See also Microorganisms,
        2:63–65
Fungi, 2:64
    abscess caused by, 2:4
    pneumonia caused by, 2:73
Fungicides, 8:7
"Funny bone," 1:35
Furnace inspection, 8:22
Furnaces, solar, 8:84

Gallbladder, 1:42–43, 42, 3:58, 81.
    See also Digestive system, 1:30–33;
    Liver, 1:60–62
Gallstones, 1:32, 42–43, 3:58–59, 58.
    See also Digestive system, 1:30–33;
    Jaundice, 3:81
Gametes, 6:40
Gamma globulin, 2:39, 43, 3:62
Gamma rays, 8:73
Gangrene, 3:10, 15, 59, 76
    frostbite and, 8:43
    See also Circulatory system,
        1:25–27; Arteriosclerosis, 3:15;
        Diabetes, 3:46–48
Gang violence, 8:92
Garlic, benefits of, 4:88–89
Gas, excessive, 3:105
Gaseous pollutants, 8:9
Gastric ulcers, 3:114
Gastritis, 3:106
Gastroenterologists, 9:33
Gastrointestinal tract, alcohol abuse
    and effect on, 7:9
Gay. See Homosexuality
Gender identity, 5:90, 6:38–40
    transsexuality and, 6:99
Gender roles, 5:90
Gene(s), 1:22, 5:50, 6:40, 41
    dominant, 6:41
    recessive, 3:42, 91, 6:41
    single mutant, birth defect due
        to, 6:11
General adaptation syndrome (GAS),
    5:96
General anesthesia, 3:13
General anesthetic, 7:17, 9:4

General (family) practitioners
    (G.P.'s), 9:32
Generalized anxiety disorder, 5:10
Generalized convulsive seizures
    (GCS), 3:54, 54
Generalized nonconvulsive seizures
    (GNCS), 3:54
Generativity versus stagnation, 5:36
Generic drugs, 7:52, 59–60. See also
    Clinical drug trials, 7:37
Gene splicing, 8:44
Gene therapy, 6:42, 8:44, 45
Genetic counseling, 3:42, 50, 75, 91,
    102, 110
Genetic counselor, 9:12. See also Ge-
    netics, 6:40–42; Genetic screening,
    6:42–44
Genetic disorders
    inheritance of, 6:41–42
    mutations causing, 6:63
    types of, 6:11
Genetic engineering, 3:80, 6:42,
    8:44–45, 9:22. See also Birth de-
    fects, 6:11–12; Genetics, 6:40–42;
    Genetic screening, 6:42–44; Med-
    ical ethics, 9:21–22
Geneticists, 6:42
Genetic predisposition, 6:11
Genetics, 1:23, 25, 6:40–42
    breakthroughs in, 6:42
    inheritance of genetic disorders,
        6:41–42
    sex determination, 6:40
    See also Cell, 1:22–23; Heredity
        and environment, 5:49–50; Ge-
        netic engineering, 8:44–45
Genetic screening, 6:11, 42–44
    amniocentesis, 6:43, 43, 78, 100
    chorionic villus sampling,
        6:43–44, 78, 100
    other techniques, 6:44
    ultrasound during, 6:43, 100
    See also Down syndrome,
        3:49–50; Hemophilia, 3:74–75
Genital herpes. See Herpes, genital
Genital infections, chlamydial, 2:20
Genital thrush, 2:19
Genital warts, 2:40, 99, 100, 6:94. See
    also Sexually transmitted diseases
    (STDs), 2:82; Syphilis, 2:87–88
Geriatrics, 9:13
Geriatric specialists, 9:33
German measles. See Rubella
Germs. See Microorganisms
Gerontologist, 9:13
Gestalt therapy, 5:80–81
Giardia lamblia, 2:69
Giardiasis, 2:69
Gigantism, 3:60

Gingivae, 1:29, 65, 99
Gingivitis, 1:29, 65, 99, 3:62, 7:36
Gland(s), 1:43
    adrenal, 1:6–7
    endocrine system of, 1:35–37
    mammary, 4:18, 6:13, 14, 34
    parathyroid, 1:36, 97
    parotid, 1:86
    pineal, 1:79
    pituitary, 1:79–80
    prostate, 1:83, 6:53
    salivary, 1:86
    sebaceous, 1:45, 89, 3:4, 4
    sweat, 1:39, 89, 2:15–16
    swollen, 1:64
    thymus, 1:54
    thyroid, 1:96–97
    See also Hormone(s), 1:51–52;
      Metabolism, 1:64–65; Dia-
      betes, 3:46–48
Glans, 6:54
Glaucoma, 3:55, 60, 83. *See also* Eye,
    1:39–41; Cataracts, 3:35–36; Dia-
    betes, 3:46–48; Eye tests, 3:55
Global warming, 8:45–46
    air pollution and, 8:9
    carbon dioxide and, 8:21
    effects of, 8:46
    energy conservation and reduc-
      tion of, 8:34
    fossil fuels and, 8:40
    as global problem, 8:46
    greenhouse effect, 8:45–46, 45
    See also Solar energy, 8:83–84
Glomerulonephritis, 2:87
Glomerulus, 1:57
Glottis, 1:30, 96
Glucagon, 1:77, 4:67
Glucose, 4:14, 15, 35, 66–67, 106,
    111
    in urine, 1:100
    See also Liver, 1:60–62; Pancreas,
      1:76–77; Diabetes, 3:46–48;
      Body metabolism, 4:15–17; Di-
      gestion, 4:32–33; Energy, food,
      4:35–36; Energy, physical,
      4:36–38; Insulin, 7:68
Glycogen, 4:35, 66
Goiter, 1:97, 3:112, 4:96
Golfer's elbow, 1:35
Gonorrhea, 2:41–42, 82, 6:94. *See*
    also Bacterial infections, 2:13–15;
    Chlamydial infections, 2:20–21;
    Nonspecific urethritis, 2:67; Pelvic
    inflammatory disease (PID),
    2:70–71
"Goosebumps," 5:16
Gout, 1:42, 3:17, 58
    low-purine diet for, 4:32

Government
    energy conservation promoted
      by, 8:34
    environmental groups in, 8:35
    hazardous waste disposal and, 8:49
Grafts, skin, 3:97
Grain alcohol. *See* Alcohol
Grains. *See* Breads and cereals group
Grand mal seizures, 3:54, 54
Grantly Dick-Read method, 6:65
Granulocytes, 1:13
Grass. *See* Marijuana
Graves' disease, 3:112
Gray matter, 1:93
Greenhouse effect, 8:45–46, 45
Greenpeace, 8:35
Greenstick fracture, 8:42
Grief
    over death and dying, 5:40–41
    over loss (other than death),
      5:37, 41
Ground fault circuit interrupter
    (GFCI), 8:30–31, 78
Groundwater, 8:94
Group dates, 6:28
Group medical care, 9:13
    clinic and, 9:6–7
    See also Physicians (M.D.'s),
      9:31–34
Group pressure, conformity to,
    5:28–29
Group programs for quitting smok-
    ing, 7:86–87
Group therapy, 5:81
Group weight-loss programs, 4:130
Growth, 1:43–44
    child development and, 1:24–25
    See also Adolescence, 1:5–6;
      Adulthood, 1:8; Aging, 1:9;
      Hormone(s), 1:51–52;
      Lifestyle, 4:71–72
Growth disorders, 3:60–61. *See also*
    Pituitary gland, 1:79–80; Malnutri-
    tion, 4:73–75
Growth hormone (GH), 1:36, 80,
    3:60, 61
Growth regulators, 4:7
Growth spurt, adolescent, 6:84
Guillain-Barré syndrome, 3:61–62.
    See also Immune system, 1:52–55;
    Nervous system, 1:71–74
Guilt, 5:43
    initiative versus, 5:35
Gum disease, 3:45, 62–63. *See also*
    Dental problems, 3:44–45; Dental
    care, 9:7–8
Gums (gingivae), 1:29, 65, 99
Gun control, 8:46–47, 93. *See also*
    Homicide, 8:53–54

Gynecological examination, 6:44–45
    Pap test, 6:69
    See also Sexually transmitted dis-
      eases (STDs), 2:82, 6:94–95;
      Infertility, 6:50–51
Gynecologist, 6:44, 9:33

Hair, 1:45–46, 45
    dandruff and, 3:43
    infection of hair roots (boil),
      2:15–16
Hair follicles, 3:4, 4
Hair loss, 1:46, 3:63–64, 63
    minoxidil to treat, 7:75
Hair transplants, 3:64
Halitosis, 1:65, 3:45
Hallucinations, 5:48
    in bereaved person, 5:40
    drug therapy for, 5:39
    psychosis and, 5:78
    schizophrenia and, 5:48, 86
    See also Delirium tremens, 7:42;
      Hallucinogens, 7:60–61; With-
      drawal syndrome, 7:100–101
Hallucinogens, 5:48, 7:51, 60–61, 84
    LSD, 7:70–71
Halothane, 7:17
Hammer (malleus), 1:33, 34
Hamstring muscles, 1:58
Hand, 1:46–47, 47
    carpal tunnel syndrome and,
      3:34–35, 35
    nails on, 1:69
    See also Arthritis, 3:15–17
Handgun Control, Inc., 8:47
Hangnails, 1:69
Hangover, 7:8, 61–62
    from sleeping pills, 7:90
    See also Withdrawal syndrome,
      7:100–101
Hansen's disease. *See* Leprosy
Happiness, 5:48–49
Hard hats, 8:78
Hard palate, 1:65
Harvard Medical School definition of
    death, 1:28
Hashish, 7:71
"Hassles"
    coping with, 5:4, 4
    as stressors, 5:96
Hay fever, 2:84, 3:6, 64–65
    treatment of, 7:25
    See also Antihistamines and
      decongestants, 7:25–27
Hazardous waste, 8:47–49, 93
    common wastes and their effects,
      8:47–48, 48

government and individual action on, 8:49
lead, 8:56
methods of dealing with, 8:48
radioactive waste, 8:48–49, 62, 73
toxic substances as, 8:91–92
HCG (human chorionic gonadotropin), 6:72
HDL cholesterol, 4:5, 23
Headache, 3:65–66
migraine, 3:88–89
See also Aneurysm, 3:13–14; Brain tumor, 3:25–26; Hypertension, 3:77–78
Head louse, 2:57, *57*
Health Care Financing Administration, 9:8
Health-care system, 9:13–14
clinics, 9:6–7
health maintenance organizations (HMOs), 9:17
rising costs of health care, 9:14, *14*, 16–17
in U.S., 9:13–14
Health-care workers, 9:14–15
emergency medical technician (EMT), 9:10–11
home health services, 9:17–18
medical technologists and technicians, 9:15, 22–23
nursing, 9:24–25
occupational therapists, 9:26–27
physical therapists, 9:30–31
podiatrist, 9:34
in speech therapy, 9:40–41
See also Eye care, 9:11–12; Physicians (M.D.'s), 9:31–34
Health educator, 9:15–16
Health insurance, 9:16–17
Medicare and Medicaid, 9:23
national health-care program, 9:17
paying for, 9:14
types of coverage, 9:16–17
See also Health-care system, 9:13–14; Health maintenance organization (HMO), 9:17
Health maintenance organization (HMO), 9:17
physician assistants in, 9:31
Health psychology, 5:44, 49
Health Resources and Services Administration, 9:9
Hearing aids, 3:67
Hearing impairments, access for people with, 8:4
Hearing loss, 1:34, 3:66–67
noise pollution and, 8:59, 79

See also Ear infections, 2:32–34; Rubella, 2:78–79
Heart, 1:47–49, *48*, 3:70
alcohol abuse and effect on, 7:9
cardiac muscle, 1:67
and circulatory system, 1:26
cycle, 1:48, *49*
electrocardiogram of, 3:51–52, *52*
heart rate, 4:68
strength of, 4:49
valves, 1:48, 49, 3:70, 73
See also Aorta, 1:11; Blood, 1:12–14; Atherosclerosis, 3:19–20; Stroke, 3:106–8
Heart attack, 1:27, 3:15, 19, 24, 68–69, *68*
aspirin and, 7:30
beta-blockers and, 7:32
CPR and, 8:24–25
See also Atherosclerosis, 3:19–20; Blood clot, 3:24; Diabetes, 3:46–48; Electrocardiogram (ECG or EKG), 3:51–52; Hypertension, 3:77–78
Heartburn, 1:32, 3:105, 106
Heart defects, 1:23
Heart disease, 1:9, 49, 67, 3:34, 69–72, 8:9
breathing difficulties caused by, 2:17
congestive heart failure, 3:17, 34, 68, 70, 71–72
coronary artery disease, 3:34, 68, *68*, 69, 70
endocarditis, 2:34–35
excess body fat and, 4:15
hypertensive, 3:34, 70
rheumatic fever, 2:77–78
stress and, 5:97
See also Rubella, 2:78–79; Aerobic exercise 4:4–6; Cholesterol, 4:23–24; Fitness, 4:48–49; Beta-blocker, 7:32
Heart-lung machine, 3:73
Heart murmur, 3:34, 72–73. *See also* Endocarditis, 2:34–35
Heart rate, 1:49, 4:5, 68
target range, 4:6, 68
See also Aerobic exercise, 4:4–6; Fitness, 4:48–49; Fitness training, 4:49–50; Running, 4:95–96; Sports and fitness, 4:99–101
Heart surgery, 3:73–74, 109
heart transplant, 3:72, 73–74
valve surgery, 3:73
See also Heart, 1:47–49
Heat cramps, 4:101

Heat exhaustion, 4:101
Heat rash, 2:76
Heatstroke, 4:101–2, 8:49–50, 99. *See also* First aid, 8:38–39
Height, growth disorder and, 3:60–61
Height and weight chart, 4:125, *125*
Heimlich, Henry, 8:50
Heimlich maneuver, 1:96, 8:24, 39, 50–51, *50*. *See also* CPR, 8:24–25
Helmets, use of, 8:14, 58
Hematologists, 9:33
Hematology, 9:29
Hemiplegia, 3:95
Hemochromatosis, 3:38
Hemodialysis, 3:49
Hemoglobin, 1:13, 14
anemia and, 3:11
iron in, 4:69
Hemoglobin S, 3:102
Hemolytic anemia, 3:12, 102
Hemophilia, 1:14, 3:74–75
AIDS and hemophiliacs, 2:4
gene therapy for, 8:44
See also Genetic screening, 6:42–44; Genetic counselor, 9:12
Hemorrhage, 8:18
cerebral, 3:107
See also Bleeding, 8:18–19
Hemorrhoids, 1:11, 3:75, *75*. *See also* Anus, 1:10–11; Rectum, 1:81
Hepatic artery, 1:61
Hepatic portal vein, 1:61
Hepatitis, 1:61, 2:42–43, 4:58
chronic, 2:43
cirrhosis and, 3:38
drug-induced, 2:43
gamma globulin to prevent, 2:39
risk factors, 2:42
type A, 2:12, 42, 43
type B, 2:42–43, *42*
See also Jaundice, 3:81
Herbicides, 8:7, 69
Heredity and environment, 5:49–50
and aging, 1:8, 9
and child development, 1:25
differences in intelligence and, 5:54
Duchenne muscular dystrophy and, 3:91
genetic disorders and, 6:41–42
and growth, 1:44
risk factors involving, 4:94–95
Tay-Sachs disease and, 3:110
See also Genetics, 6:40–42
Hernia, 3:76, *76*
Herniated ("slipped") disk, 1:94, 3:21–22

Heroin, 7:62–63, 77
    drug rehabilitation for users of,
        7:5, 16, 49–50, 63, 74
    effects of, 7:62–63
    risks of, 7:63
    withdrawal symptoms from,
        7:62–63, 101
    See also AIDS, 2:4–8; Addiction,
        7:4–5; Drug interaction,
        7:47–48; Drug overdose,
        7:48–49; Methadone, 7:74–75;
        Narcotics, 7:76–78
Herpes, genital, 2:44, 6:94
    condoms to protect against,
        6:22–23
Herpes infections, 2:44–45, 98
    acyclovir for, 7:29
    blisters of, 3:23
    nonspecific urethritis, 2:67
    See also Sexually transmitted dis-
        eases (STDs), 2:82
Herpes simplex, 1:65
Herpes simplex virus type 1, 2:97
    cold sore caused by, 2:23, 44
    encephalitis caused by, 2:34
Herpes simplex virus type 2, 2:44
Herpes zoster virus, 2:19. *See also*
    Shingles, 2:83–84
Heterosexuality, 6:45–46. *See also*
    Gender identity, 6:38–40; Sex
    roles, 6:85–86
Hiatal hernia, 3:76
Hiccups, 1:30, 3:76–77
Hierarchy of needs, 5:87, 87
High blood pressure. *See*
    Hypertension
High-density lipoprotein (HDL), 4:23
    HDL cholesterol, 4:5, 23
High-intensity laser, 3:83
Hinge joints, 1:9–10, 34–35, 46, 55,
    56, *56*, 58–59, 91
Hip, 1:50, *50*, 77
    pelvis, 1:77
    See also Connective tissue,
        1:27–28; Joint, 1:56; Musculo-
        skeletal system, 1:68–69;
        Arthritis, 3:15–17
Hippocratic oath, 9:29
Histamines, 3:6, 64, 4:53, 7:25
Histrionic personality disorder, 5:71
HIV, 1:14, 54, 2:5, 45–46, 3:25, 33,
    75, 87
    antibodies to, 2:6
    AZT to fight, 7:31
    diagnosing, 2:7--8, 46
    method of attacking cells,
        2:45–46
    preventing infection by, 2:7–8,
        46

    testing for, 2:6, 46
    transmission of, 2:5, 7–8, 46,
        6:8
    See also Immune system,
        1:52–55; AIDS, 2:4–8; Pneu-
        monia, 2:72–73; Safer sex,
        6:82–83
HIV antibody testing, 2:6, 46
Hives (urticaria), 1:90, 3:6
HMO. *See* Health maintenance orga-
    nization (HMO)
Hodgkin's disease, 3:77, 87. *See also*
    Lymphatic system, 1:63–64; Lym-
    phoma, 3:87
Holistic medicine, 9:4
Holmes, Thomas, 5:4, 96
Home delivery, 6:65
Home health aides, 9:18
Home health services, 9:17–18. *See*
    also Health-care workers, 9:14–15;
    Nursing, 9:24–25; Occupational
    therapist, 9:26–27; Physical thera-
    pist, 9:30–31
Homeopathy, 9:4
Home safety, 8:51–53
    accidents and, 8:5, 6, 51–53, 67
    for children, 8:6, 53, 68, 69
    electrical, 8:30–31, 52, 78
    equipment for, 8:77–78
    fires and, 8:52–53, 77
    household falls and, 8:51–52
    poisoning and, 8:5, 67–69, *68*
    sanitation and, 8:81
    See also Access for people with
        disabilities, 8:4–5; Burns,
        8:20–21; First aid, 8:38–39;
        Poison-Control Centers,
        8:66–67
Homicide, 8:53–54, *53*
    spouse abuse ending in, 8:86, 92
    See also Gun control, 8:46–47;
        Violence, 8:92–93
Homologous chromosomes, 6:40
Homosexuality, 6:45, 46–48
    in adolescence, 1:6
    AIDS and, 2:4
    causes of, 6:47–48
    early homosexual behavior,
        6:46–47
    marriage and, 6:56
    myths about, 6:47
    sexual practice and relationships,
        6:47
    See also Prejudice, 5:72–74; Self-
        image, 5:89–90; Bisexuality,
        6:12–13; Gender identity,
        6:38–40; Sex roles, 6:85–86
Honey, 4:111
Hookworms, 2:69

Hormonal imbalances, infertility and,
    6:50–51
Hormonal methods of contraception,
    6:24
Hormone(s), 1:51–52
    of adrenal glands, 1:6, 7, 38–39,
        51
    body metabolism and, 4:15, 16
    of endocrine glands, 1:35–37
    epinephrine, 1:38–39
    follicle-stimulating, 1:*51*, 80,
        6:84
    growth, 1:36, 80, 3:60, 61
    growth regulators mimicking,
        4:7
    of pancreas, 1:36, *51*, 77
    of pituitary gland, 1:35, 36, *51*,
        80
    sex, 1:5–6, 7, 6:84–85
    of thyroid gland, 1:*51*, 96–97
    thyroid-stimulating, 1:36, *51*, 80
    trophic, 1:35
    See also Gland(s), 1:43; Metabo-
        lism, 1:64–65; Thyroid dis-
        orders, 3:112; *specific hormones*
Hormone replacement therapy
    (HRT), 6:49, 7:63–64
Hormone therapy, 7:63–64
    for cancer, 3:31
    See also Contraception, 6:24–26;
        Endometriosis, 6:31–32; Infer-
        tility, 6:50–51; Menopause,
        6:58–59; Sex hormones,
        6:84–85; Drugs and sports,
        7:52–53
Hospice, 1:28, 9:18–19. *See also*
    Dying and bereavement, 5:40–41
Hospital, 9:19–20
    clinics attached to, 9:6–7
    history of, 9:20
    modern, 9:20
    rehabilitation centers in, 9:39
    See also Hospice, 9:18–19; Nurs-
        ing home, 9:25
Hospital emergency rooms, 8:32
Hospital social worker, 9:18
Host, of pathogen, 2:25, 50
Host factors in agent-host-environ-
    ment model, 7:57
Hot flashes, 6:58
Hot lines, 5:31
    suicide-prevention, 5:100
Hot-weather emergencies, 8:99–100
Household products used as in-
    halants, 7:66
Human bites, 8:16
Human chorionic gonadotropin
    (HCG), 6:72
Human growth hormone, 1:*51*

Human immunodeficiency virus. *See* HIV

Humanistic psychology, **5:**77

Humanistic theories of personality, **5:**70, 87

Humanistic therapies, **5:**80–81

Humerus, **1:**34, 87, 88

Hunger, **4:**8, 68–69. *See also* Hypothalamus, **1:**52

Hurricanes, **8:**100

Hyaline cartilage, **1:**27

Hydrocarbons, **8:**92
  chlorinated, water polluted with, **8:**96, *96*
  in fossil fuels, **8:**40

Hydrogenation, **4:**46

Hydrostatic weighing, **4:**14, 126–27

Hygiene, feminine, **6:**34–35, 60

Hymen, **6:**33

Hyperactivity, **5:**50–51
  Ritalin to treat, **7:**87
  See also Mind, **5:**62–63; Psychotherapy, **5:**79–82; Sleep problems, **5:**93–94

Hyperglycemia, **3:**46, **4:**67, **7:**68

Hyperopia, **3:***116*, 117

Hypertension, **1:**11, 15–16, 27, 49, 58, **3:**77–78, *78*
  cardiovascular diseases and, **3:**13, 15, *20*, 34, 70, *71*
  portal, **3:**38–39
  sodium in diet and, **4:**98
  stress and, **5:**97
  treatment of, **7:**27, 32, 44, 75
  See also Blood pressure, **1:**14–16; Kidney disorders, **3:**82–83; Stroke, **3:**106–8; Stress-management techniques, **5:**98–99; Beta-blockers, **7:**32

Hypertensive heart disease, **3:**34, 70

Hyperthyroidism, **1:**97, **3:**112

Hypertrophic scar, **1:**87

Hyperventilation, **2:**17, **3:**79

Hypnosis, **5:**51–52
  to quit smoking, **7:**87

Hypnotics. *See* Sedatives

Hypochondria, **5:**52, 79. *See also* Anxiety disorders, **5:**10–12; Psychosomatic disorders, **5:**78–79

Hypodermic syringe, **7:**67

Hypoglycemia, **1:**43, **3:**48, **4:**67, **7:**68

Hypothalamus, **1:**19, 35, *51*, 52, 79–80, **5:**42
  sense of hunger and, **4:**69
  See also Brain, **1:**19–21; Hormone(s), **1:**51–52; Nervous system, **1:**71–74

Hypothermia, **8:**54–55. *See also* Frostbite, **8:**43

Hypothyroidism, **1:**43, 65, 97, **3:**112

Hysterectomy, **6:**48–49, *48*
  endometriosis and, **6:**32, 48
  See also Cancers of the sex organs, **6:**17–18; Contraception, **6:**24–26; Menstruation, **6:**59–61

Hysteria, **5:**53. *See also* Neurosis, **5:**65; Psychosomatic disorders, **5:**78–79

Ibuprofen, **7:***16*, 28

Ice, treating injury with, **8:**76–77, *76*

Identical siblings, **6:**62, *62*

Identification, **5:**13, 29
  with peers, **5:**67–68

Identity
  adult, **5:**4–5
  gender, **5:**90, **6:**38–40
  self-image and, **5:**89–90
  versus role confusion, **5:**35

Identity crisis, **5:**90

Idiosyncratic side effects, **7:**89

Idoxuridine, **7:**29

Ileitis. *See* Crohn's disease

Ileum, **1:**32

Ilium, **1:**77

Illegal drugs. *See* Drugs and the law

Immune serum globulin. *See* Gamma globulin

Immune system, **1:**13, 52–55
  allergies and, **3:**6
  antibiotic treatment and, **2:**9
  autoimmune disorder and, **3:**20
  bacterial infections and, **2:**14
  chronic fatigue syndrome and, **3:**38
  of fetus, **6:**38
  fighting microorganisms, **2:**64–65
  Guillain-Barré syndrome and, **3:**61–62
  HIV and destruction of, **2:**45
  immunity and, **2:**47
  inflammation and, **2:**51
  maternal, breast-feeding and, **6:**14
  prevention of communicable disease by, **2:**26
  rejection of transplant, **3:**73, 113
  response to infection, **2:**50
  shingles and weakness of, **2:**83
  stress and, **5:**44, 97
  viral infection and, **2:**97–98
  See also AIDS, **2:**4–8; Antibody(ies), **2:**10; Antigen, **2:**10–11; Fever, **2:**37–38; Immunization, **2:**47–49; Immunotherapy, **3:**79–80

Immunity, **2:**47
  antiserum and, **2:**11–12
  natural, **1:**54, **2:**47
  as response to infection, **2:**50
  types of, **2:**47, 48
  See also Immune system, **1:**52–55; Antibody(ies), **2:**10; Antigen, **2:**10–11; Gamma globulin, **2:**39; Immunization, **2:**47–49; Interferon, **2:**53–54

Immunization, **1:**54, *54*, 55, **2:**47–49
  active, types of, **2:**48
  antibodies stimulated by, **2:**10
  against communicable disease, **2:**26
  flu shots, **2:**53
  functioning of, **2:**47–48
  for poliomyelitis, **2:**73, 74
  reactions to and risks of, **2:**48–49
  recipients of active, **2:**49
  schedule of, **2:**48, *49*
  for smallpox, **2:**85
  for tetanus, **2:**90
  for viral infections, **2:**98
  for whooping cough, **2:**100
  See also Immune system, **1:**52–55; Antibody(ies), **2:**10; Antiserum, **2:**11–12

Immunodeficiency diseases, **1:**54
  AIDS, **2:**4–8

Immunologists, **9:**33

Immunosuppressants, **1:**55, **7:**65
  opportunistic infections and, **2:**68
  See also Immune system, **1:**52–55; Autoimmune disorder, **3:**20; Transplant surgery, **3:**113; Corticosteroids, **7:**40

Immunotherapy, **1:**54–55, **3:**7, 31–32, 79–80. *See also* Immune system, **1:**52–55; Genetic engineering, **8:**44–45

Impacted teeth, **3:**45

Impetigo, **1:**90, **2:**49–50, 57
  blisters of, **3:**23

Implant, drug, **7:**83

Implantation of zygote, **6:**36

Impotence, **6:**89

Incentives, **5:**64

Incest, **6:**49–50. *See also* Family, **5:**44–45; Child abuse, **8:**22–23

Incineration, **8:**48, 85

Incision, **8:**101

Incisors, **1:**99, *99*

Incomplete proteins, **4:**76, 90

Incontinence, **3:**80. *See also* Diabetes, **3:**46–48; Multiple sclerosis, **3:**89–90; Stroke, **3:**106–8

Incubation period of infection, **2:**50

Incubator for premature babies, 6:77
Incus (anvil), 1:33, 34
Independent emergency centers, 9:6
Indigestion (dyspepsia), 3:105
    acid, 7:18
    See also Stomachache/indiges-
        tion, 3:105–6
Indirect-action anticoagulants, 7:23
Industrial and organizational psy-
    chology, 5:77
Industrial effluent, 8:91
Industrial smog, 8:82
Industry
    particulates from, 8:66
    recycling in, 8:76
    water pollution caused by, 8:95,
        96
Industry versus inferiority, 5:35
Infancy, 1:24, 43
Infantile paralysis. See Poliomyelitis
Infatuation, 5:59
Infection, 2:50–51
    abscess and, 2:4
    antibiotic ointment to reduce risk
        of, 7:20
    antiseptics to prevent, 7:28–29
    bacterial, 2:13–15
    body's response to, 2:50
    boil, 2:15–16
    burns and, 8:20
    chlamydial, 2:20–21
    fever and, 2:37–38
    fungal, 2:38–39
    herpes, 2:44–45
    opportunistic, 2:67–68
    parasitic, 2:68–69
    salmonella, 2:80
    secondary, 7:21
    sources of, 2:51
    stages of, 2:50–51
    streptococcal, 2:86–87
    viral, 2:97–98
    See also Antibody(ies), 2:10;
        Antigen, 2:10–11; Communi-
        cable diseases, 2:24–26; Immu-
        nity, 2:47; Microorganisms,
        2:63–65
Infectious arthritis, 3:17
Inferiority, industry versus, 5:35
Infertility, 6:50–51. See also Adop-
    tion, 6:6–7; Endometriosis,
    6:31–32; Female reproductive sys-
    tem, 6:33–34; Miscarriage,
    6:61–62; Pregnancy, 6:74–76; Sex
    hormones, 6:84–85
Infestation, 2:68
Inflammation, 2:51–52
    anti-inflammatory drugs to re-
        duce, 7:28

of bronchi, 2:17–18
development of, 2:51
inflammatory response, 1:53, 53
as response to infection, 2:50
treatment of, 2:52
See also Immune system,
    1:52–55; Antibody(ies), 2:10;
    Conjunctivitis, 2:26–27; Fever,
    2:37–38; Arthritis, 3:15–17;
    Autoimmune disorder, 3:20
Inflammatory bowel disease, 3:39
Influenza, 1:85, 2:52–53
    pandemic of 1918–1919, 2:36
    See also Immune system, 1:52–55
Influenza virus, 2:97, 97
Informational communication, 5:23
Informed consent, 9:29
Ingredients, list of, 4:56, 71
Ingrown toenail, 1:69, 3:57
Inguinal hernia, 3:76
Inhalants, 7:51, 65–66, 84. See also
    Drugs and the law, 7:53–54; Drug
    use and abuse, 7:55–57
Inhalation of drugs, 7:56
Inheritance of genetic disorders,
    6:41–42
Initiative versus guilt, 5:35
Injection, 7:56, 67
    insulin, 7:68, 68
    See also AIDS, 2:4–8; Drug use
        and abuse, 7:55–57
Injuries, 8:55–56
    bites and stings, 8:15–18
    bleeding from, 8:18–19
    burns, 8:20–21
    caused by fire, 8:36
    dislocations, 8:26
    electrical, 8:52
    fractures, 8:41–43
    frostbite, 8:43
    on the job, 8:79
    minor, first aid for, 8:38
    RICE technique for, 8:76–77, 76,
        87
    sports, 4:102–5
    sprains and strains, 8:86–88
    wounds, 8:101
    See also Rabies, 2:75; Child
        abuse, 8:22–23; Violence,
        8:92–93
Inner ear, 1:33, 34, 3:67
Insanity, 5:61
Insect bites and stings, 8:16–17, 55
Insecticides, food contamination by,
    4:58
Insect repellent, 7:67–68
Insects, food contamination by, 4:62
Insight, 5:30
Insoluble fibers, 4:47

Insoluble proteins, 4:91
Insomnia, 1:92, 3:103, 5:93
Instincts, 5:63
Instrumental conditioning. See Oper-
    ant conditioning
Insulin, 1:51, 77, 3:46, 48, 7:68
    blood sugar level and, 4:67
    diabetes and, 3:46–48
    hormone therapy with, 7:64
    injection of, 7:68, 68
    pancreas and production of,
        1:76–77, 7:68
Insulin-dependent diabetes mellitus
    (IDDM), 3:46, 47, 48
Insurance, health. See Health
    insurance
Integration, 1:72
Integrity versus despair, 5:36
Intellectual development, 5:34–35,
    57
Intellectual health, 5:60
Intelligence, 5:53–54
    definitions of, 5:53–54
    differences in, 5:54
    mental retardation and, 5:62
    testing, 5:54
Intensive care unit, 9:20
Intercostal muscles, 1:23
Intercourse, sexual. See Sexual
    intercourse
Interferon, 2:53–54, 98, 7:22
    as defense against viruses, 2:63
    See also Immune system, 1:52–55;
        Viral infections, 2:97–98; Ge-
        netic engineering, 8:44–45
Intermediate-care facility (ICF), 9:25
Intermediate lobe (pituitary), 1:80
Internal bleeding, 8:18–19
Internalization, 5:13, 29
International Olympic Committee,
    7:52, 94
Internists, 9:33
Internship, 9:32
Interstitial fluid, 1:98
Intestines. See Colon; Digestive sys-
    tem; Small intestine
Intimacy, 5:54, 83
    marital, 6:55
    versus isolation, 5:35–36
Intoxication, 7:7–8, 68–69
    legal, defined, 7:9, 33, 46, 68
Intramuscular injections, 7:67
Intrauterine device. See IUD
Intravenous injections, 7:67
Intravenous (IV) drug use, AIDS and,
    2:4
In vitro fertilization, 6:51, 9:22
Involuntary muscles, 1:67
Iodine, 1:97, 4:80, 80, 96

Ionizing radiation, 8:72, 73
Ions, 8:72
Ipecac, syrup of, 8:69
IQ. *See* Intelligence
IQ tests, 5:54, 62
Iris, 1:39, 40
Iron, 4:69–70, 80, *80*
Iron deficiency, 4:69–70, 114
Iron-deficiency anemia, 3:11–12, 4:70
Irradiation, 4:60
Irritable-bowel syndrome, 2:30
Ischium, 1:77
Islets of Langerhans, 1:36, 77
Isokinetic exercise, 4:108
Isolation, intimacy versus, 5:35–36
Isometric exercise, 4:108
Isotonic exercise, 4:108, 132
Isotretinoin (Accutane), 7:19
Itching, 2:54
  eczema and, 3:51
  scabies and, 2:81
  See also Skin, 1:89–90; Fungal
    infections, 2:38–39; Parasitic
    infections, 2:68–69; Rash,
    2:76–77
IUD, 6:24, 25, *25*, 51–52, *52*
  pelvic inflammatory disease and,
    2:70, 71, 6:52
  See also Contraception, 6:24–26;
    Female reproductive system,
    6:33–34

James, William, 5:76
James-Lange theory of emotion, 5:42,
  43
Jarvik-7 artificial heart, 3:74
Jaundice, 1:61, 3:38, 81, *81*
  hepatitis A and, 2:42
  See also Liver, 1:60–62; Malaria,
    2:59–60
Jaw, 1:55, *55*, *68*, 91
  temporomandibular joint syn-
    drome and, 3:110–11
  See also Mouth, 1:65–66; Skull,
    1:91; Tooth, 1:99–100
Jealousy. *See* Emotion
Jejunum, 1:32
Jellyfish stings, 8:17–18
Jenner, Edward, 2:47, 85
Jet lag, 1:92
Job safety. *See* Safety on the job
Jock itch, 2:39, 7:25
Johnson, Virginia, 6:93
Joint(s), 1:56
  ankle, 1:9–10
  ball-and-socket, 1:50, 56, *56*, 77,
    87–88

of big toe, bunion on, 3:57
elbow, 1:34–35
hinge, 1:9–10, 34–35, 46, 55, 56,
  56, 58–59, 91
hip, 1:50
inflammation of. *See* Arthritis
injuries, 1:56
knee, 1:58–59
in musculoskeletal system, 1:68
pivot, 1:56, 70
sacroiliac, 1:77
shoulder, 1:87–88
sprains involving, 8:86–88, *87*
temporomandibular, 1:55, 3:*110*
wrist, 1:46
See also Connective tissue,
  1:27–28; Arthritis, 3:15–17
Joy, 5:48
Jugular veins, 1:70
Juices, 4:11–12
Junk food, 4:70–71. *See also* Fast
  food, 4:43; Fats, oils, and sweets
  group, 4:46–47; Food labeling,
  4:56–57; Recommended dietary allowance (RDA), 4:92–93; Snack
  food, 4:97
Justifiable homicide, 8:54
Juvenile rheumatoid arthritis, 3:17

Kaposi's sarcoma, 2:5, 6, 3:81–82
  AIDS and, 2:46, 3:81–82
  See also Immune system,
    1:52–55
Keloid scar, 1:87
Keratin, 1:45, 69
Keratoses, 8:88
Kidney, 1:57–58, *57*
  and excretory system, 1:39
  and urinary tract, 1:101
  See also Adrenal glands, 1:6–7;
    Enzyme, 1:37–38; Hyperten-
    sion, 3:77–78
Kidney disorders, 3:82–83
  dialysis and, 3:48–49
  See also Diabetes, 3:46–48; Hy-
    pertension, 3:77–78; Shock,
    3:101
Kidney failure, 3:48–49, 82–83
Kidney stones, 1:58, 101, 3:82, *82*
Kidney transplant, 3:83
Killed-virus vaccines, 2:48
Kilocalorie, 4:20
Kinsey, Alfred, 6:12
Kinsey Scale of Sexual Orientation,
  6:*12*
Kissing, HIV transmission and "wet"
  (deep, French, tongue), 2:8, 46

Kissing disease. *See* Mononucleosis
Knee, 1:58–59, *58*
  injuries, 4:103, *103*
  sprained, 8:87
  See also Connective tissue,
    1:27–28; Musculoskeletal sys-
    tem, 1:68–69
Knee-jerk reflex, 1:81
Kohlberg, Lawrence, 5:36
Kübler-Ross, Elisabeth, 5:40
Kwashiorkor, 4:73–74

Labeling
  of antihistamines and deconges-
    tants, 7:26
  and drug interaction warnings,
    7:48
  of food, 4:56–57
Labia majora and labia minora, 1:83,
  6:33
Labor, 6:75
  premature, 6:75
  stages of, 6:20–21, 64
Laboratory technologists and techni-
  cians, medical, 9:22–23
Laboratory tests, 1:78
Labyrinth (inner ear), 1:34
Laceration, 4:103–4, 8:101
Lactic acid, 4:7
Lactoovovegetarians, 4:113
Lactose, 4:111
Lactose intolerance, 4:54, 78, 111
Lactovegetarians, 4:113
Laetrile, 9:37
Laissez-faire leaders, 5:55
Lamaze method, 6:21, 65
Landfills, 8:85
Lanugo, 4:33
Laparoscope, 3:58, 6:32, 51
Laparoscopy, 2:70, *70*, 6:32, 51
Large intestine. *See* Colon
Laryngitis, 1:96, 2:54–55. *See also*
  Throat, 1:95–96
Larynx, 1:70, 84, 95, 96, 2:55
Laser surgery, 3:83
Late adulthood, 1:8
Latissimus dorsi muscles, 1:88
Law(s)
  drugs and, 7:53–54, 55
  gun control, 8:47
  right-to-die, 9:21
  tobacco and, 7:98–99, 8:60–61
  traffic, 8:12, 14
Laxatives, 3:41, 4:27, 7:69–70, 73.
  See also Diarrhea, 2:29–30; Dehy-
  dration, 4:26–27; Fiber, 4:47–48
Lazarus, Richard, 5:96
LDL cholesterol, 4:23, 24

L-dopa, 3:96, 7:70. *See also* Parkinson's disease, 3:95–96
Leaching fields, 8:82
Lead, 8:*48*, 56, 91. *See also* Air pollution, 8:9–10; Hazardous waste, 8:47–49; Particulates, 8:65–66; Toxic substances, 8:91–92
Leadership, 5:55
Learning, 5:56–57
    to be responsible, 5:85
    cognitive, 5:57
    of concepts, 5:24–25
    conditioning, 5:25–27, 56
    factors affecting, 5:57
    intelligence and, 5:53
    modeling, 5:56–57
    observational, 5:85
    See also Developmental psychology, 5:34–36; Motivation, 5:63–64
Learning disability, 5:58
Leboyer method, 6:65
Legionnaires' disease, 2:55–56
Legumes, 4:76, 107
Lens, 1:39, *40*
    cataracts in, 3:35–36, *35*
    implants, 3:36
    vision problems and, 3:116, *116*
Leprosy, 2:56–57
Lesbians, 6:46. *See also* Homosexuality, 6:46–48
Lethal dose, 7:45
Leukemia, 1:18, 3:83–84, *84*, 113. *See also* Blood, 1:12–14; Bone marrow, 1:18–19; Anemia, 3:11–12; Immunotherapy, 3:79–80
Leukocytes. *See* White blood cells (leukocytes)
Levodopa (L-dopa), 3:96, 7:70
LH (luteinizing hormone), 1:80, 6:84
Lice, 2:57, 96
Licensed practical nurse (L.P.N.) (licensed vocational nurse), 9:25
Life changes, coping with major, 5:4, *4*
Life expectancy, 1:59–60. *See also* Lifestyle, 4:71–72
Life jackets, use of, 8:27, 99
Life span, 1:60
Lifestyle, 4:71–72
    and blood diseases, 1:14
    and blood pressure, 1:16
    cancer prevention and, 3:32
    communicable diseases and, 2:26
    as controllable risk factor, 4:95
    coronary artery disease treatment and, 3:69
    diet and, 4:30–32
    early adulthood and choice of, 1:8
    exercise and, 4:40

    and growth, 1:44
    and heart disease, 1:49
    hypertension treatment and, 3:78
    and kidney problems, 1:58
    and life expectancy, 1:60
    and physical examination, 1:78
    rest and, 4:93–94
    sedentary, 3:19, *20*, 71
    stress and, 5:29, 97
    weight management and, 4:132
    wellness and, 4:133
Life-support systems, 3:41
    medical ethics of, 9:21
Ligaments, 1:27
    in ankle, 1:10
    in elbow, 1:34
    in foot, 1:41–42
    in hip joint, 1:50
    in mouth, 1:65
    periodontal, 1:99
    in shoulder, 1:88
    sprains involving, 8:86–88, *87*
Lightning, dangers of, 8:31, 100
Lingual frenulum, 1:65
Lipids, 4:14–15
Lipoproteins, 4:23
Liposuction, 3:97, 4:72. *See also* Plastic surgery, 3:97; Body composition, 4:13–14
Lips, 1:65
Liquid diets, 4:42
Lisping, 3:104
Listener, being a good, 5:23
Lithium, 5:39
Liver, 1:39, 60–62, *60*
    alcohol abuse and effect on, 7:9
    hepatitis and inflammation of, 2:42–43
    yellow fever and damage to, 2:101
    See also Digestive system, 1:30–33; Gallbladder, 1:42–43
Liver biopsy, 3:38, 81
Liver disease
    cancer, 3:33
    cirrhosis, 3:38–39
    jaundice as symptom of, 3:81
Live-virus vaccines, 2:48
Living wills, 9:21, 29
Lobotomy, 5:82
Lobules, liver, 1:61, *61*
Local anesthetic, 3:12–13, 7:17, 67, 9:4
Lockjaw. *See* Tetanus
Look-alike drugs, 7:70. *See also* Antihistamines and decongestants, 7:25–27; Drug interaction, 7:47–48; Drugs and the law, 7:53–54

"Looking-glass self," 5:90
Loperamide, 7:24
Love, 5:58–59
    companionate, 5:59
    divorce and, 5:36–37
    happiness and, 5:48
    intimacy and, 5:54
    marriage and, 6:55–56
    romantic, 5:36, 59
    sexual attraction and, 6:87–88
Low-density lipoprotein (LDL), 4:23
    LDL cholesterol, 4:23, 24
Low-impact aerobics, 4:6
Low-intensity laser, 3:83
Low-salt (low-sodium) diet, 4:31, 98–99
LSD, 7:61, 70–71. *See also* Hallucinogens, 7:60–61
Lubricant laxatives, 7:69
Lumbar puncture, 2:58, *58*
    encephalitis diagnosis and, 2:34
    meningitis diagnosis and, 2:62
    See also Spinal cord, 1:93–94
Lumbar vertebrae, 1:94
Lumpectomy, 3:27, 6:56
Lung, 1:39, 62–63, *62*, 84
    aerobic exercise and, 4:5
    breathing difficulties and, 2:16–17
    cystic fibrosis and, 3:42–43
    See also Circulatory system, 1:25–27; Respiratory system, 1:84–86
Lung cancer, 1:85, 3:85
    marijuana and, 7:73
    radon exposure and, 8:74
    smoking and, 2:36–37, 3:85
    See also Tobacco, 7:97–99; Radon, 8:74
Lung disease, 3:85–87
    asthma, 3:17–19
    bronchitis, 2:17–18
    chronic obstructive, 2:18
    emphysema, 3:53
    lung cancer, 3:85
    particulates and, 8:65–66
    pleurisy, 3:98
    pneumonia, 2:72–73
    tuberculosis, 2:95
Lunula, 1:69
Lupus erythematosus, 3:87
Luteinizing hormone (LH), 1:80, 6:84
Lyme disease, 2:58–59. *See also* Arthritis, 3:15–17
Lymph, 1:64
Lymphatic system, 1:63–64, *64*
    adenoids, 1:4–5
    metastasis through, 3:27, 29, *29*
    tonsils, 1:98

See also Immune system, 1:52–55; Hodgkin's disease, 3:77; Lymphoma, 3:87

Lymph nodes, 1:63, 64, 70

Lymphocyte, 1:13, 53, 64, 2:5, 97
immunosuppressants and, 7:65

Lymphoma, 3:87. *See also* Lymphatic system, 1:63–64; Opportunistic infections, 2:67–68; Hodgkin's disease, 3:77

Lysergic acid diethylamide (LSD), 7:61, 70–71

M.D.'s. *See* Physicians (M.D.'s)

Macrobiotic diet, 4:72, 73, *73. See also* Diets, 4:30–32; Fad diets, 4:42–43

Macrolides, 7:21

Macrominerals, 4:79

Macronutrients, 4:21, 45, 82, 83, *83,* 90
carbohydrates, 4:21–22
fats, 4:45–46
proteins, 4:90–92

Macrophages, 1:13

Macular degeneration, 3:55

Magnesium, 4:79, *80*

Magnetic resonance imaging (MRI), 3:*26,* 88, *88,* 8:73. *See also* CAT scan, 3:36; X-ray examination, 3:117–18

Mainlining, 7:62

Mainstream smoke, 7:92

Maintenance stage of relationship, 5:83

Major depression, 5:33–34

Major medical insurance, 9:16

Major tranquilizers, 5:39, *39*

Malaria, 2:25, 59–60, 69
spread of, 2:59, *59*
symptoms and diagnosis of, 2:60
treatment and prevention of, 2:60

Male pattern baldness, 3:63, *63*

Male reproductive system, 1:82, 83, 6:52–54, *53*
ejaculation and, 6:54, 67, 84, 91, 93
erection and, 6:54
passage of sperm through, 6:53–54
production of sperm in, 6:52–53
See also Fertilization, 6:35–37; Female reproductive system, 6:33–34; Testicular self-examination, 6:98–99

Male sex hormones, 6:84–85

Male sexual dysfunction, 6:88–89

Malignant melanoma, 3:102

Malignant tumor, 3:29, 114

Malleus (hammer), 1:33, *34*

Malnutrition, 3:36, 61, 4:73–75. *See also* Anemia, 3:11–12; Eating disorders, 4:33–34; Nutrition, 4:84–85; Underweight, 4:113

Malocclusion, 3:45, 92

Malpractice, 9:29

Mammary glands, 4:18, 6:13, 14, 34

Mammogram, 3:26, 28, 118, 6:45, 54–55, *54*
breast cancer detection with, 3:26–28
See also Mastectomy, 6:56–57

Mandible, 1:55

Manganese, 4:*80,* 81

Mania, 5:18, 34

Manic-depressive illness. *See* Bipolar disorder

Manipulation of dislocated bone, 8:26

Manslaughter, 8:54

Manubrium, 1:24

Marasmus, 4:74

Marijuana, 7:51, 71–73. *See also* Addiction, 7:4–5; Drugs and the law, 7:53–54; Drug use and abuse, 7:55–57; Hallucinogens, 7:60–61; Psychoactive drugs, 7:84–85

Marriage, 6:55–56
alternatives to, 6:56, *56*
divorce and, 5:36–37
sex and love in, 5:58–59, 6:55–56
See also Adult identity, 5:4–5; Family, 5:44–45; Intimacy, 5:54

Marriage therapy, 5:81

Marrow. *See* Bone marrow

Maslow, Abraham, 5:77, 87

Masochism, 6:9

Mass hysteria, 5:53

Mastectomy, 3:27, 6:56–57, *57*
breast cancer and, 3:26–28
breast implants after, 6:15
See also Chemotherapy, 3:37; Radiation therapy, 3:99; Tumor, 3:114; Anticancer drugs, 7:22–23; Hormone therapy, 7:63–64

Master gland. *See* Pituitary gland

Masters, William, 6:92

Mastoiditis, 2:34

Masturbation, 6:57–58
orgasm and, 6:67–68
prevention of STDs with, 6:95
safer sex through, 6:57, 83
sexual fantasies and, 6:90

Maxilla, 1:55

Maxillary sinuses, 1:89

Maximum heart rate, 4:68

Maximum life span, 1:60

Meals-on-Wheels, 9:18

Measles, 2:36, 60–61
MMR vaccine for, 2:61, 66, 79
See also Encephalitis, 2:34; Pneumonia, 2:72–73

Meats, eggs, and legumes group, 4:50, 51, 64, *64,* 75–77. *See also* Heart disease, 3:69–72; Dietary guidelines, 4:28–29; Exchange system, 4:38–39; Food group systems, 4:55–56

Meat thermometer, using, 4:62

Median nerve, 3:34, *35*

Mediator, conflict resolution and, 5:27

Medical care, 9:13–14

Medical degrees, types of, 9:31–32

Medical emergencies, 8:38

Medical ethics, 9:21–22
abortion and, 6:4–5
clinical drug trials and, 7:37
genetic engineering and, 8:44–45
transplant surgery and, 3:113

Medical examiner, 2:13

Medical history, 1:78
in gynecological examination, 6:44

Medical insurance. *See* Health insurance

Medical research and testing, 9:22

Medical self-care, 8:56–57. *See also* First aid, 8:38–39; Home health services, 9:17–18

Medical technologists and technicians, 9:15, 22–23. *See also* Anesthesiologist, 9:4–5; Physicians (M.D.'s), 9:31–34; Radiologist, 9:38–39; Surgeon, 9:41

Medicare and Medicaid, 9:14, 23
administration of, 9:8
home health services covered by, 9:18
hospice program included in, 9:19
Medicare A and Medicare B, 9:23
nursing home care covered by, 9:25
See also Health-care system, 9:13–14; Health insurance, 9:16–17

Medicinal drugs, 7:51–52

Medicine, genetic engineering in, 8:44

Medicine cabinet, 7:73–74, *74*
first aid supplies in, 8:38
See also Drug interaction, 7:47–48; Drugs, 7:50–52; Drug use and abuse, 7:55–57

Meditation, 4:94, 5:18, 84, 99
Medulla (brain), 1:19
Medulla (hair), 1:45
Meiosis, 1:23
Melanin, 1:45, 89, 8:88
Melanocyte-stimulating hormone (MSH), 1:80
Melanoma, 1:90, 3:102
Melatonin, 1:79
Meltdown, 8:62
Membrane, cell, 1:22
Memory loss, amnesia and, 5:6–7
Men
    cancers of sex organs in, 6:17–18
    fertility testing of, 6:51
    hormone therapy for, 7:64
    infertility in, 6:50
    sexual dysfunction among, 6:88–89
Menarche, 1:5, 6:59, 79
Ménière's disease, 3:67
Meninges, 2:61, 62
Meningitis, 1:74, 93, 2:61–62, 62
    cerebral palsy and, 3:37
Menopause, 1:18, 84, 6:58–59, 61, 85
    bone loss in women after, 3:93
    hormone replacement therapy and, 7:63
    See also Female reproductive system, 6:33–34
Menstrual cycle, 6:59–60, 59, 85
    cravings during, 4:54
Menstruation, 1:5, 64, 84, 6:33, 59–61
    birth-control pill use and, 6:10
    end of, 6:58, 61
    feminine hygiene during, 6:34–35, 60
    irregular periods, 6:60–61
    menstrual cycle, 6:59–60, 59, 85
    premenstrual syndrome and, 6:60, 77–78
    puberty and menarche, 6:59, 79
    See also Toxic shock syndrome, 2:92–93; Endometriosis, 6:31–32; Fertilization, 6:35–37
Mental health, 5:59–60. See also Communication, 5:22–23; Coping skills, 5:29–30; Responsibility, 5:84–85; Self-actualization, 5:87; Self-esteem, 5:88–89
Mental illness(es), 5:60–61
    antisocial personality, 5:9
    bipolar disorder, 5:18–19
    classifying, 5:60–61, 61
    depression, 5:32–34

multiple personality, 5:64–65
    paranoia, 5:66–67
    personality disorders, 5:70–71
    psychosis, 5:78
    psychotherapy for, 5:79–82
    treating, 5:61
Mental retardation, 5:62, 62
    cerebral palsy and, 3:36
    Down syndrome and, 3:49–50
    See also Heredity and environment, 5:49–50; Intelligence, 5:53–54; Learning disability, 5:58; Genetics, 6:40–42
Meperidine, 7:16, 77
Mercury poisoning, 8:48, 91, 96
Mescaline, 7:61
Mesmer, Franz Anton, 5:51
Metabolism, 1:7, 64–65, 4:66
    of alcohol, 7:6
    basal metabolic rate, 1:64–65, 4:15–16, 37–38, 37
    body, 4:15–17
    See also Hormone(s), 1:51–52; Pancreas, 1:76–77; Thyroid gland, 1:96–97
Metacarpal bones, 1:46, 3:35
Metastasis, 3:26, 27, 27, 30, 30, 114
Metastatic tumor, 3:25
Metatarsals, 1:41
Methadone, 7:16, 74–75, 77
    drug rehabilitation using, 7:16, 50, 74
    See also Drug overdose, 7:48–49; Narcotics, 7:76–78
Methyl alcohol, 7:6
Methylphenidate. See Ritalin
Michigan Alcoholism Screening Test, 7:13, 14
Microminerals, 4:79
Micronutrients, 4:82, 83, 84
    minerals, 4:79–81
    vitamins, 4:121–22
Microorganisms, 2:63–65
    blood test for, 1:16
    culture of, 2:28–29
    fighting against, 2:64–65
    food spoilage and, 4:59
    types of, 2:63–64, 63
    See also Immune system, 1:52–55; Antibiotic treatment, 2:8–10; Antigen, 2:10–11; Bacterial infections, 2:13–15; Candida infections, 2:19; Communicable diseases, 2:24–26; Fungal infections, 2:38–39; Immunization, 2:47–49; Parasitic infections, 2:68–69; Viral infections, 2:97–98

Microsurgery, 3:109
Midbrain, 1:19
Middle adulthood, 1:8, 5:5
Middle ear, 1:33, 34, 3:67
    infections of, 2:32–33
Midgets, 3:61
Midwife, 9:14, 24
Migraine headache, 3:66, 88–89, 91. See also Stress-management techniques, 5:98–99; Beta-blockers, 7:32
Milk, breast, 4:18–19, 6:13, 14, 14
Milk and milk products group, 4:12, 50, 51, 64, 64, 77–78. See also Heart disease, 3:69–72; Dietary guidelines, 4:28–29; Exchange system, 4:38–39; Food group systems, 4:55–56
Mind, 5:62–63
    unconscious, 5:31, 63
    See also Sleep, 1:91–92; Central nervous system, 5:20–21; Emotion, 5:42–44; Perception, 5:68; Drug use and abuse, 7:55–57
Minerals, 4:65, 77, 79–81, 80, 83, 84
    calcium, 4:19–20
    iron, 4:69–70
    potassium, 4:89
    sodium, 4:97–99
    See also Body metabolism, 4:15–17; Nutrients, 4:82–84; Vitamins, 4:121–22
Mini-pill, 6:10
Minor depression, 5:33
Minority groups, prejudice against, 5:72, 73
Minor tranquilizers, 5:39, 39
Minoxidil, 3:64, 7:75. See also Hair loss, 3:63–64
Miscarriage, 6:4, 61–62, 75
    signs of, 6:61, 61
    See also Abortion, 6:4–5; Female reproductive system, 6:33–34
Mistrust, trust versus, 5:35
Mites, 2:81, 96
Mitochondrion (mitochondria), 1:23
Mitosis, 1:23, 6:30
MMR (measles, mumps, rubella) vaccine, 2:61, 66, 79
Modeling, 5:56–57. See also Role model, 5:85
Modified radical mastectomy, 6:57
Molars, 1:99
Molds, 2:64
Molybdenum, 4:80, 81
Mono. See Mononucleosis
Monoamine oxidase inhibitors (MAOIs), 7:23, 24

Monocytes, 1:13
Monogamy, mutual, 6:83, 95
Mononucleosis, 2:65, 3:38
Monosaccharide, 4:107, 110, 111
Monosodium glutamate (MSG), 4:52,
    53, 82, 98. See also Food additives,
    4:52–53; Salt, 4:96–97
Monounsaturated fats, 4:46, 46
Mons (mons pubis, mons veneris),
    6:33
Mood, alcohol's effect on, 7:8
Mood disorders, 5:33–34
Mood swings, suicide and, 5:100
Moral development, 5:36
Morning sickness, 2:98, 6:74
Morphine, 7:16, 62, 77
Mosquitoes, diseases spread by
    malaria, 2:25, 59, 60, 69
    yellow fever, 2:25, 101
Mothers Against Drunk Driving
    (MADD), 7:47
Motion sickness, 8:57–58, 58
Motivation, 5:63–64
    self-actualization and, 5:87
    See also Learning, 5:56–57;
        Prosocial behavior, 5:74
Motorcycle safety, 8:6, 58. See also
    Accidents, 8:5–6; Automobile
    safety, 8:11–13
Motor neurons, 1:74, 81, 93
Motor vehicle accidents, 8:5, 12, 13.
    See also Automobile safety,
    8:11–13
Mouth, 1:65–66, 66, 86
    cold sore on, 2:23
    See also Dental examination,
        1:29; Mucous membrane, 1:66;
        Salivary glands, 1:86; Tooth,
        1:99–100; Dental problems,
        3:44–45; Gum disease,
        3:62–63
Mouth-to-mouth resuscitation, 8:24,
    25, 27, 31, 38
Mouthwash, 7:76. See also Dental
    problems, 3:44–45; Dental care,
    9:7–8
MSG, 4:52, 53, 82, 98
Mucous membrane, 1:52, 65, 66, 76
    diphtheria and infection of,
        2:30–31
    in nasal passages, 1:66, 76
    warts on, 2:99–100
Mucus, 1:31, 66, 76, 88
    cervical, 6:66, 68
    in lungs, bronchitis and, 2:17,
        18
Mucus method of family planning,
    6:66
Multifactorial disorders, 6:11

Multifactorial inheritance, 6:42
Multiple birth, 6:36, 62–63. See also
    Fertilization, 6:35–37; Premature
    baby, 6:76–77
Multiple orgasms, 6:67
Multiple personality, 5:64–65
Multiple sclerosis, 1:74, 93, 3:89–90.
    See also Nervous system, 1:71–74;
    Autoimmune disorder, 3:20
Mumps, 1:86, 2:65–66
    MMR vaccine for, 2:61, 66, 79
Murder, 8:54, 93
Murmur, heart, 3:34, 72–73
Muscle biopsy, 3:23
Muscle cells, 1:22
Muscle paralysis, 3:95
Muscles, 1:66–67, 88
    aerobic exercise and, 4:5
    body building and, 4:12–13
    cardiac, 1:67
    hamstring, 1:58
    intercostal, 1:23
    latissimus dorsi, 1:88
    Parkinson's disease and, 3:96
    quadriceps, 1:58
    sore, 4:104
    sphincter, 1:10
    strains of, 3:21, 8:86–88
    trapezius, 1:88
    triceps, 1:34, 35, 67, 67
    See also Connective tissue,
        1:27–28; Musculoskeletal sys-
        tem, 1:68–69; Muscular dys-
        trophy, 3:90–91
Muscle strength, 4:48–49
Muscle tissue, 1:98
Muscular dystrophy, 1:67, 3:90–91.
    See also Birth defects, 6:11–12; Ge-
    netic screening, 6:42–44; Genetic
    counselor, 9:12
Muscular endurance, 4:34, 35, 49,
    99, 100
Musculoskeletal system, 1:68–69, 68.
    See also Connective tissue,
    1:27–28; Exercise, 4:39–40
Mutagens, 6:64
Mutation, 6:41, 63–64
    of single genes, birth defects
        from, 6:11
    See also Genetics, 6:40–42
Mutual monogamy, 6:83, 95
Myasthenia gravis, 1:67
Myelin, 1:93
Myelin sheath, 3:62, 89, 90
Myocardial infarction. See Heart
    attack
Myocarditis, 3:71
Myocardium, 1:47
Myofibrils, 1:66

Myoglobin, 4:69
Myopia, 3:116–17, 116

Nails, 1:46, 69, 69. See also Hair,
    1:45–46; Skin, 1:89–90; Fungal in-
    fections, 2:38–39; Foot problems,
    3:57–58
Narcissistic personality disorder, 5:71
Narcolepsy, 1:92, 3:103, 104, 7:15, 87
Narcotics, 3:94, 7:51, 76–78, 84
    analgesics, 7:15–16, 16
    antidiarrheal drugs, 7:24
    athletes' abuse of, 7:53
    designer, 7:43
    effects of, 7:77
    risks of, 7:77–78
    types of, 7:77
    withdrawal symptoms from,
        7:77, 101
    See also AIDS, 2:4–8; Addiction,
        7:4–5; Drug overdose, 7:48–49;
        Drug rehabilitation, 7:49–50;
        Drugs and the law, 7:53–54;
        Drug use and abuse, 7:55–57;
        Heroin, 7:62–63; Injection,
        7:67; Methadone, 7:74–75;
        Withdrawal syndrome,
        7:100–101
Nasal cavity, 1:91
Nasal decongestants, 7:26–27
Nasal passages, 1:75–76
    adenoids in, 1:4, 5
    mucous membranes in, 1:66, 76
National Cancer Institute, 4:10, 89
National Center for Health Statistics,
    9:8
National Cholesterol Education Pro-
    gram, 4:24
National health-care program, 9:17
National Institutes of Health (NIH),
    4:129, 9:9, 9
National Interagency Council on
    Smoking and Health, 8:60
National Library of Medicine, 9:9
National Priority List (NPL) of Super-
    fund program, 8:89, 89, 90
National Rifle Association (NRA), 8:47
National Weather Service, 8:100
Natural childbirth, 6:20, 21, 64–65.
    See also Apgar test, 6:8–9; Cesarean
    section, 6:19; Female reproductive
    system, 6:33–34; Fetus, 6:37–38;
    Miscarriage, 6:61–62; Placenta,
    6:71–72; Prenatal care, 6:78; Nurs-
    ing, 9:24–25
Natural family planning, 6:5, 24, 25, 66
    abstinence and, 6:5
    contraception and, 6:24–26

See also Female reproductive system, 6:33–34; Sexual intercourse, 6:91–92

Natural food. *See* Organic food

Natural gas, 8:40

Natural immunity, 1:54, 2:47

Nature versus nurture. *See* Heredity and environment

Navel, 6:101

Near-drownings, 8:26

Nearsightedness, 3:116–17, *116*

Neck, 1:70. *See also* Respiratory system, 1:84–86; Spinal cord, 1:93–94; Throat, 1:95–96; Thyroid gland, 1:96–97

Needle biopsy, 3:22, 26–27

Needs, hierarchy of, 5:87, *87*

Negative emotion, 5:42

Negative reinforcement, 5:26, 56

Neglect, parental, 8:23

Negotiation, conflict resolution and, 5:27

Neisseria gonorrhoeae, 2:41, *41*

Neologisms, 5:86

Neomycin, 7:20

Neonatal care unit, 6:77

Neonatal conjunctivitis, 2:27

Neonatal jaundice, 3:81

Neoplasm. *See* Tumor

Nephritis, 3:82

Nephrologists, 9:33

Nephron, 1:57

Nerve blocks, 3:13

Nerve cells, 1:22, 89

Nerve damage, 1:75

Nerves, 1:71, 75
 median, 3:34, *35*
 olfactory, 1:76
 optic, 1:40
 parasympathetic, 1:73
 pinched, 1:74, 75
 sensory, 3:94
 sympathetic, 1:73
 vestibulocochlear, 3:67

Nerve tissue, 1:98

Nerve transplants, 3:95

Nervous system, 1:71–74, *72*
 autonomic, 5:15–16
 brain and, 1:19–21
 central, 5:20–21
 endocrine stimulation by, 1:35–36
 paralysis and damage to, 3:95
 parasympathetic, 5:15, 16, *16*
 Parkinson's disease and, 3:95–96
 perception and, 5:68
 peripheral, 1:71, 73, *73*, 5:15, 20
 proteins and regulation of, 4:91
 somatic, 1:73
 spinal cord and, 1:93–94

Neuralgia, 3:91. *See also* Shingles, 2:83–84

Neurologists, 1:74, 9:33

Neuron, 1:74–75, *74*, 3:53
 main types of, 1:71–72, *74*, 81, 93
 See also Brain, 1:19–21

Neuropsychiatry, 5:75

Neuropsychology, 5:77

Neurosis, 5:60, 65. *See also* Anxiety, 5:9–10; Anxiety disorders, 5:10–12; Depression, 5:32–34; Hypochondria, 5:52; Mental illness, 5:60–61; Psychosis (psychotic disorder), 5:78

Neurotransmitters, 1:74, 7:15, 95

Newborns
 Apgar test for, 6:8–9, *8*
 premature, 6:76–77, 98
 See also Childbirth, 6:20–21

Niacin, 4:*116*, 117, *121*

Nicotine, 7:86, 91, 92, 96
 addictive nature of, 7:85
 in chewing tobacco and snuff, 7:36
 withdrawal symptoms from, 7:101

Nicotine skin patches, 7:87

Night blindness, 3:54

Nightmares, 5:38, 94

Night terrors, 5:94

Nipple, 6:13

Nitrites, 4:52, 53

Nitrogen oxides, 8:91
 in acid rain, 8:7, *7*, 9–10

Nitrous oxide, 7:17, 66

Nocturnal emission, 6:54, 67, 80. *See also* Male reproductive system, 6:52–54

Noise pollution, 8:59–60, 79. *See also* Ear, 1:33–34; Hearing loss, 3:66–67

Nongonococcal urethritis. *See* Nonspecific urethritis

Non-Hodgkin's lymphoma, 3:87

Non-insulin-dependent diabetes mellitus (NIDDM), 3:46, 47, 48

Nonionizing radiation, 8:72, 73

Nonnarcotic analgesics, 7:15, *16*, 17

Nonprescription drugs, 7:52, 78–79
 antacids, 7:18–19
 antibiotic ointment, 7:20
 antihistamines and decongestants, 7:25–27
 aspirin, 7:30
 cough medicine, 7:41
 FDA review of, 7:59
 generic, 7:60
 guide to use of, 7:*79*

 laxatives, 7:69–70
 nonnarcotic analgesics, 7:*16*, 17
 side effects of, 7:79, 89
 sleeping pills, 7:90
 See also Clinical drug trials, 7:37; Drug allergy, 7:47; Prescription drugs, 7:82–83

Nonpsychotic disorders, 5:60, 65

Non-REM sleep, 1:91, 92

Nonsmokers' rights, 8:60–61

Nonspecific urethritis, 2:20, 67. *See also* Urinary tract, 1:100–101; Chlamydial infections, 2:20–21; Herpes infections, 2:44–45

Nonsteroidal anti-inflammatory drugs (NSAIDs), 7:28

Nonverbal communication. *See* Body language

Norepinephrine, 1:7

Norms, 5:100

Norplant, 6:26

Nose, 1:75–76, *75*
 rhinoplasty on, 3:97
 See also Adenoids, 1:4–5; Respiratory system, 1:84–86; Common cold, 2:23–24

Nosebleed, 1:76, 3:91–92, *92*. *See also* Hemophilia, 3:74–75; Hypertension, 3:77–78

Nose drops. *See* Antihistamines and decongestants

Notochord, 6:30

Nuclear family, 5:44

Nuclear medicine technologists, 9:23

Nuclear power, 8:61–62
 radioactive waste from, 8:48–49, 62, 73
 See also Solar energy, 8:83–84

Nuclear reactor, 8:61

Nucleus (cell), 1:22

Numbness, bereavement and sense of, 5:40

Nurse anesthetists, 9:4, 5, 24. *See also* Anesthesiologist, 9:4–5

Nurse midwife, 9:24

Nurse practitioner, 9:24

Nurses' aide, 9:25

Nursing, 9:24–25. *See also* Healthcare workers, 9:14–15; Home health services, 9:17–18; Physicians (M.D.'s), 9:31–34; Surgeon, 9:41

Nursing home, 9:25
 rehabilitation center at, 9:39

Nutrients, 4:82–84, *83*
 added to foods, 4:52
 from breads and cereals, 4:17
 from breast milk, 4:18, 19
 carbohydrates, 4:21–22

diet and supply of, **4**:30
digestion and, **4**:32
fats, **4**:45–46
from fruits and vegetables, **4**:65–66
from meats, eggs, and legumes group, **4**:76–77
from milk and milk products, **4**:77
minerals, **4**:79–81
proteins, **4**:90–92
RDA of, **4**:*80*, 92–93, *121*, 122
vitamins, **4**:121–22
Nutrition, **4**:84–85
malnutrition, **4**:73–75
stress prevention and, **5**:29
See also Cancer, **3**:29–32; Diabetes, **3**:46–48; Heart disease, **3**:69–72; Hypertension, **3**:77–78; Body metabolism, **4**:15–17; Nutrients, **4**:82–84; Phytochemicals, **4**:88–89
Nutritional therapy, **4**:85
Nutritionist, **4**:85, **9**:26
Nutrition labeling, **4**:56–57, *57*

Obesity, **4**:85–86, 128
breathing difficulties caused by, **2**:17
disease and, **3**:19, *20, 71*
overweight and, **4**:87
See also Body metabolism, **4**:15–17; Diet aids, **4**:27–28; Diet foods, **4**:29–30; Diets, **4**:30–32; Risk factors, **4**:94–95; Weight assessment, **4**:124–27; Weight management, **4**:130–32
Oblique fracture, **8**:*42*
Observational learning, **5**:85
Obsessions, **5**:11
Obsessive-compulsive disorder, **5**:11–12
Obstetrician/gynecologists, **6**:44, **9**:33
Obstructive breathing disorder, **2**:17
Occipital lobe, **1**:21
Occupational medicine, **9**:35
Occupational Safety and Health Administration (OSHA), **8**:62–63. *See also* Accidents, **8**:5–6; Asbestos, **8**:10–11; Environmental organizations, **8**:35; Fire safety, **8**:36–37; Lead, **8**:56; Safety equipment, **8**:77–79; Safety on the job, **8**:79–80; Toxic substances, **8**:91–92
Occupational therapist, **9**:26–27. *See also* Home health services, **9**:17–18; Physical therapist, **9**:30–31

Occupation-related lung diseases, **3**:86–87
Ocean dumping, **8**:85, 97
Office of Human Development Services, **9**:8
Oils. *See* Fats, oils, and sweets group
Oil spills, **8**:40, 63–64. *See also* Fossil fuels, use of, **8**:40–41; Toxic substances, **8**:91–92
Older adulthood, **5**:5
Olecranon ("funny bone"), **1**:35
Olfactory nerve, **1**:76
Oncologists, **9**:33
OPDs (outpatient departments), **9**:6, 20
Open adoption, **6**:6
Open fracture, **8**:41, 42
Open-heart surgery, **3**:73
Operant conditioning, **5**:25, 26–27, *26, 56*
Operations. *See* Surgery
Ophthalmic surgery, **3**:109
Ophthalmologist, **3**:55, **9**:11, 33
Ophthalmoscope, **3**:55
Opiate receptors, **1**:37, **7**:16
Opiates, **7**:16, 77
Opioids, **7**:77
Opportunistic infections, **2**:67–68
AZT and, **7**:31
HIV infection and, **2**:5, 6, 7, 46
See also Immune system, **1**:52–55; Candida infections, **2**:19; Herpes infections, **2**:44–45; Autoimmune disorder, **3**:20
Optician, **9**:11–12
Optic nerve, **1**:40
Optometrist, **3**:55, **9**:11, 14
Oral cancer, **7**:36
Oral contraceptive. *See* Birth-control pill
Oral sex, **6**:67, 94. *See also* Sexual intercourse, **6**:91–92
Oral surgeon, **9**:7
Oral temperature, **8**:19
Oral thrush, **2**:19
Orbits, **1**:91
Organelles, **1**:23
Organic brain disorders, **5**:61, 66
Alzheimer's disease and, **3**:9–10
brain tumor and, **3**:25–26
See also Dementia, **3**:43–44; Stroke, **3**:106–8; Senility, **5**:90–91; Delirium tremens, **7**:42
Organic food, **4**:86, **8**:8. *See also* Agricultural chemicals, **4**:6–7; Food safety, **4**:61–63; Food and Drug Administration, **7**:59; Agricultural pollution, **8**:7–8
Organ meats, **4**:75

Organ transplants, **3**:113, **9**:22
Orgasm, **6**:54, 67–68, 91, 93. *See also* Female reproductive system, **6**:33–34; Male reproductive system, **6**:52–54; Sexual dysfunction, **6**:88–89
Orthodontic devices, **3**:45, 92, 111, **9**:7–8. *See also* Dental care, **9**:7–8
Orthodontist, **3**:45, 92, **9**:7–8
Orthopedic surgery, **3**:109
Orthopedists, **4**:105, **9**:33
Orthotic devices, **4**:10, 106
Ossification, **1**:17
Osteoarthritis, **1**:18, 35, 50, 56, 59, 70, 88, **3**:15–16, 22
Osteomalacia, **1**:18, **4**:119
Osteomyelitis, **1**:18, **2**:68. *See also* Bone, **1**:17–18
Osteopathic manipulative treatment (OMT), **9**:28
Osteopathic physicians (D.O.'s), **9**:27–28, 31. *See also* Alternative health care, **9**:4; Physicians (M.D.'s), **9**:31–34
Osteopathy, **9**:28
Osteoporosis, **1**:18, 69, **3**:93, *93*, **4**:19. *See also* Calcium, **4**:19–20; Vitamin D, **4**:118–19; Menopause, **6**:58–59; Sex hormones, **6**:84–85
Otolaryngologists, **9**:33
Otosclerosis, **3**:67
Outer ear, **1**:33
infections of, **2**:32
Outpatient departments, **9**:6, 20
Ova. *See* Ovum, ova
Oval window, **1**:33, 34
Ovarian cancer, **6**:17
Ovaries, **1**:36, 83, 84, **6**:33
hysterectomy and surgical removal of, **6**:48–49
Overdose, drug. *See* Drug overdose
Overdosing, **5**:40
Overload, **4**:108, 132
Over-the-counter drugs. *See* Nonprescription drugs
Overweight, **4**:87
obesity, **4**:85–86
weight-loss strategy for, **4**:128–30
See also Weight assessment, **4**:124–27
Ovulation, **1**:5, **6**:33, 68, *68*
menopause and, **6**:58
unpredictable timing of, **6**:35
See also Abstinence, **6**:5; Contraception, **6**:24–26; Female reproductive system, **6**:33–34; Natural family planning, **6**:66; Pregnancy, **6**:74–76

Ovum, ova, **1**:83, **6**:33, 59, *59*, 68
    fertilization of, **6**:30, 33, 35–37,
        36
Oxygen–carbon dioxide exchange,
    1:12, 26, 62, 63, 84
Oxygen debt, **4**:7, 40
Oxytocin, **1**:*51*, 80, *80*
Ozone, **8**:64–65
    air pollution caused by, **8**:9
    ground-level, **8**:64
    health hazards caused by, **8**:100
    in smog, **8**:64, 90
    See also Skin cancer, **3**:102–3;
        Biosphere, **8**:14–15; Global
        warming, **8**:45–46
Ozone layer, **8**:10, 64–65, 73

Pacemaker, **1**:49, **3**:71
    artificial, **3**:74
Pain, **3**:94, *94*
    abdominal, **3**:14, 97
    anesthesia to prevent, **3**:12–13
    anesthetic drugs to block, **7**:17
    anti-inflammatory drugs for, **7**:28
    of arthritis, **3**:16
    aspirin for relief of, **7**:30
    back, **1**:94
    corticosteroids to reduce, **7**:40
    endorphins and, **1**:37
    headache, **3**:65–66
    of heart attack, **3**:68
    jaw and head, TMJ syndrome
        and, **3**:110, 111
    migraine headache, **3**:88–89
    neuralgia, **3**:91
    phantom limb, **3**:10
    of pleurisy, **3**:98
    psychological factors in, **3**:94
    of sciatica, **3**:21
    of tooth decay, **3**:44
    See also Brain, **1**:19–21; Nervous
        system, **1**:71–74; Spinal cord,
        1:93–94
Painkillers. *See* Analgesics
Pallor, **1**:89
Pancreas, **1**:36, *51*, 76–77, *76*
    blood sugar level and, **4**:67
    diabetes and, **3**:46–48
    insulin produced by, **7**:68
    See also Digestive system,
        1:30–33; Endocrine system,
        1:35–37; Cystic fibrosis,
        3:42–43; Diabetes, **3**:46–48
Pancreatic enzymes, **1**:32, 76
Pandemic, **2**:36
Panic, night terrors and, **5**:94
Panic disorder, **5**:11
Pantothenic acid, **4**:*116*, 117, *121*

Papanicolaou, G. N., **6**:69
Pap test, **2**:40, 44, **3**:32, **6**:17, 45, 69,
    69. *See also* Gynecological exami-
    nation, **6**:44–45
Para-aminobenzoic acid (PABA), **7**:97
Paralysis, **3**:95, 107
    poliomyelitis and, **2**:74
    See also Nervous system,
        1:71–74; Brain tumor, **3**:25–26;
        Multiple sclerosis, **3**:89–90;
        Muscular dystrophy, **3**:90–91;
        Stroke, **3**:106–8; Physical ther-
        apist, **9**:30–31
Paramedic, **9**:10–11
Paranoia, **5**:66–67. *See also* Drug
    therapy, **5**:39–40
Paranoid personality disorder, **5**:67,
    70
Paraplegia, **3**:95
Parasites
    foods contaminated by, **4**:58
    types of, **2**:68–69, *69*, 88–89, 91
Parasitic infections, **2**:68–69
    malaria, **2**:59–60
    treatment and prevention of, **2**:69
    trichinosis, **2**:94
    See also Immune system,
        1:52–55; Microorganisms,
        2:63–65; Anemia, **3**:11–12
Parasitic worms, **2**:64
Parasympathetic nerves, **1**:73
Parasympathetic nervous system,
    5:15, 16, *16*
Parathyroid glands, **1**:36, 97
Parathyroid hormone, **1**:*51*
Paratyphoid fever, **2**:96
Parenthood, **6**:69–71. *See also* Family,
    5:44–45; Teenage pregnancy,
    6:97–98
Parents
    adolescent conflicts with, **1**:6
    and development of children's
        self-esteem, **5**:89
    as role models, **5**:85
Parents Anonymous, **8**:23
Parietal lobe, **1**:21, **5**:21
Parkinson's disease, **1**:74, **3**:95–96
    treatment of, **7**:70
    See also Encephalitis, **2**:34; Brain
        tumor, **3**:25–26; Cardiovascular
        disease, **3**:34
Parotid glands, **1**:86
Partial seizure, **3**:53
Particulates, **8**:9, 65–66
    air pollution and, **8**:9–10
    See also Allergies, **3**:6–8; Cancer,
        3:29–32; Lung disease, **3**:85–87;
        Smoking, **7**:90–92; Lead, **8**:56;
        Safety on the job, **8**:79–80

Passive-aggressive personality dis-
    order, **5**:71
Passive exercises, **9**:31
Passive immunity, **2**:47, 48
Passive prevention of accidents, **8**:6
Passive restraints, **8**:12
Passive protection in safety equip-
    ment, **8**:77
Passive smoking, **7**:92, **8**:60
Passive solar heating systems, **8**:84
Pasta, **4**:18
Pasteurization, **4**:59
Patellar reflex, **1**:81
Pathogens, **1**:52, 53, **2**:24–25
    infection caused by, **2**:50–51
    types of, **2**:50, 64–65
Pathologist, **2**:13, **9**:28–29, 33. *See*
    also Autopsy, **2**:13
Patients' rights, **9**:29
Pavlov, Ivan, **5**:25, *25*, 77
PCBs (polychlorinated biphenyls),
    8:*48*, 92
    water polluted with, **8**:96
PCP (angel dust), **7**:61
Pediatricians, **9**:33
Pedophilia, **6**:9
Peer pressure, **5**:67–68
Pelvic examination, **6**:44, *44*, 45
Pelvic inflammatory disease (PID),
    2:70–71
    birth-control pill use and, **6**:10
    causes and treatment of, **2**:70
    gonorrhea and, **2**:41
    IUDs and risk of, **2**:70, 71, **6**:52
    nonspecific urethritis and, **2**:67
    prevention of, **2**:70
    risk factors, **2**:70, 71
    symptoms and diagnosis, **2**:70
    See also Reproductive systems,
        1:82–84; Peritonitis, **3**:97
Pelvis, **1**:50, 69, 77, *77*. *See also* Hip,
    1:50
Penicillin, **2**:9, *9*, **7**:20, 80
    for diphtheria, **2**:31
    for gonorrhea, **2**:41
    for streptococcal infections,
        2:87
    See also Antibiotic treatment,
        2:8–10; Bacterial infections,
        2:13–15; Antibiotics, **7**:20–22
Penile prostheses, **6**:89
Penis, **1**:83, **6**:53–54
    circumcision of, **6**:21–22, *22*, 54
    See also Condom, **6**:22–24
Peptic ulcer, **3**:114–15, *115*
Perception, **5**:68, *68*
    schizophrenic distortion, **5**:86
Percutaneous umbilical cord sam-
    pling, **6**:44

Pericarditis, 3:71
Pericardium, 1:47
Period. *See* Menstruation
Periodic abstinence method. *See* Natural family planning
Periodontal ligament, 1:99
Periodontitis, 1:29, 65, 99, 3:62–63
Periosteum, 1:18
Peripheral nervous system, 1:71, 73, 73, 5:15, 20
Peripheral vision, 3:55, 60
Perishable foods, 4:62
Peristalsis, 1:32
Peritoneum, 1:4
Peritonitis, 2:70, 96, 3:14, 19, 39, 97, 115
Perls, Fritz, 5:80
Pernicious anemia, 3:12
Personality(ies), 5:69–70
    adult identity and, 5:4–5
    happiness and, 5:48
    health and, 5:70
    multiple, 5:64–65
    shyness and, 5:91
    theories of, 5:69–70
    type A, 5:7, 70, 97
    type B, 5:70, 97
    See also Attitudes, 5:13–14; Psychology, 5:76–78
Personality disorders, 5:70–71
    antisocial personality, 5:9
    multiple personality, 5:64–65
    paranoid, 5:67, 70
    schizophrenia, 5:86
    schizotypal, 5:67, 70
    See also Anxiety, 5:9–10; Mental illness, 5:60–61; Psychotherapy, 5:79–82
Person-centered therapy, 5:80
Perspiration, 4:26, 87–88
    antiperspirant to reduce, 7:42
    dehydration and, 4:26, 88, 101
    sports and heat problems and, 4:101–2
    See also Beverages, 4:10–12
Pertussis. *See* Whooping cough
Pesticides, 4:7, 58, 86, 8:7, 8, 69
Petit mal seizures (absences), 3:54
Petroleum, 8:40
    products, poisoning by, 8:67, 68
Petting, 6:29
Peyote, 7:61
Phagocytes, 1:53, 54
Phalanges (foot), 1:41
Phalanges (hand), 1:46
Phantom limb pain, 3:10
Pharmacist, 9:29–30
    pharmacology and, 7:80–81
    prescription drugs and, 7:82–83

See also Drug interaction, 7:47–48; Generic drugs, 7:59–60; Nonprescription drugs, 7:78–79; Side effects, 7:89; Physicians (M.D.'s), 9:31–34
Pharmacology, 7:80–81. *See also* Dosage, 7:45–46; Drug allergy, 7:47; Drug interaction, 7:47–48
Pharyngitis. *See* Sore throat
Pharynx. *See* Throat
Phenobarbital, 7:32
Phenylketonuria, 4:9
Phenylpropanolamine (PPA), 4:27, 7:43, 44
Phlebitis, 1:102, 3:24, 34
Phlegm, 1:38
Phobia, 5:11, 11, 80
Phosphorus, 4:79, 80
Photochemical smog, 8:82
Photosynthesis, carbon dioxide and, 8:21
Physical attractiveness
    friendship and, 5:47
    sexual attraction and, 6:87–88
Physical dependence, 7:4–5, 73, 77
    on alcohol, 7:8, 14
    on sedatives, 7:88
Physical disabilities, access for people with, 8:4–5
Physical energy. *See* Energy, physical
Physical examination, 1:78–79. *See also* Dental examination, 1:29; Electrocardiogram, 3:51–52; Eye test, 3:55; X-ray examination, 3:117–18; Gynecological examination, 6:44–45; Mammogram, 6:54–55; Physicians (M.D.'s), 9:31–34
Physical growth, 1:43–44
Physical therapist, 9:30–31. *See also* Home health services, 9:17–18
Physical therapy, 3:37, 95
Physical violence, 5:5
Physician assistant (P.A.), 9:31
Physicians (M.D.'s), 9:31–34
    anesthesiologists, 3:13, 9:4–5, 33
    choosing, 9:34
    genetic counselor, 9:12
    group medical care, 9:13
    Hippocratic oath of, 9:29
    ophthalmologists, 9:11, 33
    osteopathic physicians in contrast to, 9:27–28, 31
    pathologist, 9:28–29, 33
    in preventive medicine, 9:34
    primary care, 9:32–33
    psychotherapists, 9:35–36
    radiologist, 9:34, 38–39
    specialists, 9:33–34, 41

specialties, 9:32, 32
surgeon, 9:41
See also Cancer, 3:29–32; Heart disease, 3:69–72; Kidney disorders, 3:82–83; Health-care system, 9:13–14
Physiological changes, emotions and, 5:42
Physiological cravings, 4:54–55
Phytochemicals, 4:88–89
    beta carotene, 4:10
    fiber, 4:47–48
    minerals, 4:79–81
    vitamin B complex, 4:116–17
    vitamin C, 4:117–18
    vitamin E, 4:119–20
Phytosterols, 4:89
Piaget, Jean, 5:34–35, 57
Pickling, 4:60
Pill, the. *See* Birth-control pill
Pills, 7:83
Pimples, 2:4
Pinched nerves, 1:74, 75
Pineal gland, 1:79. *See also* Circadian rhythm, 5:22
Pinkeye. *See* Conjunctivitis
Pinna, 1:33
Pinworms, 2:69
Pituitary gland, 1:7, 79–80, 6:84
    disorders of, 1:80
    and endocrine system, 1:35
    endorphins produced by, 1:37
    growth disorders and, 3:60, 61
    hormones produced by, 1:35, 36, 51, 80
    and hypothalamus, 1:52
    location of, 1:79
    puberty triggered by, 1:5, 6:79–80
    See also Growth, 1:43–44
Pivot joint, 1:56, 70
Placebo effect, quack treatments and, 9:38
Placebos, 3:9, 7:81–82. *See also* Endorphins, 1:37; Medical ethics, 9:21–22
Placenta, 6:36, 71–72, 74
    chorionic villus sampling from, 6:43, 78
    delivery of, 6:21
    development of, 6:30
    function of, 6:71–72
    multiple births and, 6:62–63
    umbilical cord and, 6:101, 101
    See also Amniotic fluid, 6:7; Childbirth, 6:20–21; Female reproductive system, 6:33–34; Miscarriage, 6:61–62; Prenatal care, 6:78

Placenta previa, 6:71, 72
Plague, 2:36, 71–72. See also Epidemic, 2:36
Plantar warts, 2:99
Plants, poisonous. See Poisonous plants
Plaque
    arterial, 1:27, 3:19, 34, 74, 107
    dental, 1:29, 65, 99, 3:44, 62, 63
    mouthwash to reduce dental, 7:76
Plasma, 1:12, 13
Plasmapheresis, 3:62
Plasmodia, 2:59, 59, 60
Plastic surgery, 3:97, 97, 109
    breast implants, 6:15
    liposuction, 4:72
    See also Surgeon, 9:41
Plateau stage of sexual response cycle, 6:93
Platelets, 1:12, 13, 18
Pleura, 1:62, 3:98
Pleurisy, 1:63, 3:98. See also Lung, 1:62–63
Pneumoconiosis, 3:86, 86
Pneumonia, 2:72–73
    asthma and, 3:18
    bacterial, 2:72, 73
    causes and diagnosis of, 2:72–73
    Chlamydia trachomatis and, 2:21
    influenza and, 2:52
    Legionnaires' disease, 2:55–56
    nonbacterial, 2:73
    Pneumocystis carinii, 2:5, 6, 46, 73
    See also AIDS, 2:4–8; Microorganisms, 2:63–65
Pneumonic plague, 2:71
Pneumothorax, 3:85–86
Podiatrist, 4:106, 9:34. See also Foot problems, 3:57–58
Poison-Control Centers, 8:66–67. See also Bites and stings, 8:15–18; Emergency care services, 8:32–33; Home safety, 8:51–53; Poisonous plants, 8:69–70; Toxic substances, 8:91–92
Poisoning, 8:67–69
    accidental, in home, 8:5, 6, 67, 68, 68
    from animal and insect bites, 8:17
    blood, 3:24–25, 101
    carbon monoxide, 8:21–22, 91
    contact, 8:67, 70
    drug overdose, 7:48–49
    first aid for, 8:68–69
    food, 4:57–58
    lead, 8:48, 56, 91

mercury, 8:48, 91, 96
    prevention of, 8:69
    sun, 8:88
    See also Air pollution, 8:9–10; Occupational Safety and Health Administration (OSHA), 8:62–63; Safety on the job, 8:79–80; Toxic substances, 8:91–92
Poisonous plants, 8:69–70, 70
    contact poisoning by, 8:67, 70
    internal poisoning by, 8:69–70
    See also Toxic substances, 8:91–92
Poisonproofing. See Home safety
Poliomyelitis, 2:73–74
Pollen, 8:66
Pollen count, 8:10
Pollution. See Agricultural pollution; Air pollution; Noise pollution; Water pollution
Pollution standards index (PSI), 8:10, 10
Polychlorinated biphenyls (PCBs), 8:48, 92, 96
Polyps
    in rectum, 1:81
    on vocal cords, 1:96
Polyunsaturated fats, 4:46, 46
Pons, 1:19
Pool safety, 8:27, 98–99
Poppers, 7:66
Population growth, 8:70–72
    dangers of uncontrolled, 8:71
    rate of, 8:71, 71
    solutions to problems of, 6:24–26, 8:71–72
    See also Air pollution, 8:9–10; Global warming, 8:45–46; Water pollution, 8:95–97
Pore, 3:4
Pornography, 6:72–73
    rape and, 6:81
    sexual fantasies and, 6:90
    See also Violence, 8:92–93
Portal hypertension, 3:38–39
Portuguese man-of-war stings, 8:17–18
Positive emotion, 5:42
Positive outlook, 5:29
Positive reinforcement, 5:17, 26, 56
Postconventional level of moral development, 5:36
Posterior lobe (pituitary), 1:80
Postgonococcal urethritis. See Nonspecific urethritis
Postherpetic neuralgia, 3:91
Posthypnotic suggestion, 5:52
Postmortem. See Autopsy

Postpartum depression, 6:73–74. See also Depression, 5:32–34
Post-traumatic stress disorder (PTSD), 5:12, 71–72. See also Anxiety disorders, 5:10–12; Crisis intervention, 5:31; Stress, 5:95–98
Pot. See Marijuana
Potassium, 4:79, 80, 89. See also Minerals, 4:79–81; Sodium, 4:97–99
Potentiation, drug, 7:48
Poultry, 4:75
Poverty, malnutrition and, 4:75
PPA (phenylpropanolamine), 4:27, 7:43, 44
Practice, 5:57
Practitioners, 9:14
    general (family), 9:32
    nurse, 9:24
Preadolescent (preteen) stage, 1:25
Pre-AIDS, 2:6
Preconventional level of moral development, 5:36
Predictable side effects, 7:89
Preeclampsia, 6:75
Pregnancy, 6:74–76
    amniocentesis during, 3:50
    amniotic fluid in uterus during, 6:7, 7, 20
    childbirth and, 6:20–21
    cocaine use during, 7:38
    contraception to prevent, 6:24–26
    cravings during, 4:54
    detecting, 6:75–76
    disorders of, 6:75
    ectopic, 2:70, 6:10, 36–37, 52, 75
    embryo and, 6:30–31
    ending, 6:4–5, 75
    fainting during, 3:56
    fertilization for, 6:35–37
    fetal alcohol syndrome and drinking during, 7:58–59
    fetus and, 6:37–38
    genetic screening during, 6:11, 42–44, 100
    heroin use during, 7:63
    malnutrition during, 3:36
    miscarriage and, 6:4, 61–62, 75
    morning sickness during, 2:98
    multiple birth, 6:36, 62–63
    myths about, 6:97
    natural childbirth and, 6:64–65
    placenta, 6:71–72
    premature baby and, 6:76–77
    prenatal care during, 6:21, 45, 63, 76, 78, 98
    preparation for breast-feeding during, 6:14
    Rh incompatibility in, 6:82

rubella during, **2:**61, 78, 79, **3:**35, 36, 67, 72, **6:**12, 75
sedative use during, **7:**88
smoking during, **7:**91
stages (trimesters) of, **6:**37–38, 74–75, *74*
teenage, **6:**97–98
ultrasound's use during, **6:**78, 100
See also Female reproductive system, **6:**33–34
Prejudice, **5:**72–74
against homosexuals, **6:**46
self-esteem and, **5:**89
Premature baby, **6:**76–77, 98. *See also* Birth defects, **6:**11–12; Childbirth, **6:**20–21; Fetus, **6:**37–38; Teenage pregnancy, **6:**97–98
Premature ejaculation, **6:**88–89
Premenstrual syndrome (PMS), **6:**60, 77–78
Premolars (bicuspids), **1:**99
Prenatal care, **6:**45, 78
genetic screening and, **6:**42–44
for multiple births, **6:**63
preparing for childbirth and, **6:**21
prevention of prematurity and, **6:**76
for teenage pregnancy, **6:**98
See also Premature baby, **6:**76–77; Rh factor, **6:**82; Fetal alcohol syndrome, **7:**58–59; Physicians (M.D.'s), **9:**31–34
Preoperational stage, **5:**35
Prepared childbirth. *See* Natural childbirth
Presbycusis, **3:**67
Presbyopia, **3:**117
Preschool stage, **1:**25
Prescription drugs, **7:**52, 82–83
antibiotics, **7:**20–22
antihypertensives, **7:**27
anti-inflammatory drugs, **7:**28
common abbreviations used with, **7:**83
contraceptive implant, **6:**26
as controlled substances, **7:**53
forms of, **7:**83
generic, **7:**60
pharmacist and preparation of, **9:**29–30
safe use of, **7:**83
used illicitly as inhalants, **7:**66
See also Drug use and abuse, **7:**55–57; Food and Drug Administration (FDA), **7:**59; Generic drugs, **7:**59–60; Nonprescription drugs, **7:**78–79
Preservatives, **4:**52, 59–60, 63

President's Council on Physical Fitness and Sports, **4:**90
sports and fitness and, **4:**99–101
See also Exercise, **4:**39–40; Fitness training, **4:**49–50
Pressure point technique, **8:**18
Preventive medicine, **4:**133, **9:**34–35. *See also* Department of Health and Human Services, **9:**8–10; Osteopathic physicians (D.O.'s), **9:**27–28; Physicians (M.D.'s), **9:**31–34
Primaquine, **2:**60
Primary care physician, **9:**32–33
Primary emotion, **5:**43
Primary hypertension, **3:**78
Primary tumor, **3:**25
Prince William Sound, oil spill in (1989), **8:**64
Prion, **2:**64
Priorities, **5:**29
Private adoptions, **6:**6
Problem solving, **5:**29
Processed meats, **4:**75
Proctoscopy, **1:**11
Proctosigmoidoscopy, **3:**40
Prodromal period of infection, **2:**50
Progesterone
in birth-control pills, **6:**9
function of, **6:**85
hormone therapy with, **7:**63–64, *64*
ovulation and, **6:**68
produced by placenta, **6:**72
Progression in weight training, **4:**132
Progressive relaxation, **4:**94, **5:**84, 99
Prohibition laws, **7:**53
Projection, **5:**32
Prolactin, **1:***51*, 80, **6:**85
Prolapse, valve, **3:**70
Prolapsed uterus, **6:**48
Pro-life and pro-choice activists, **9:**21
Pronation, **4:**10
Proof (alcohol), **7:**6
Prophylaxis, **1:**29
Propyl gallate, **4:**52
Prosocial behavior, **5:**74
Prostaglandins, **7:**15, 28, 30, 40
Prostate cancer, **6:**17–18
Prostate gland, **1:**83, **6:**53
Prosthesis, **3:**10
Protein(s), **4:**76, 83, *83*, 90–92, *91*
blood, **1:**61
enzymes, **1:**37
in urine, **1:**100
Protein-calorie malnutrition, **4:**74
Prototypes, **5:**25
Protozoans, **2:**68-69
amebic dysentery caused by, **2:**31
malaria caused by, **2:**59

nonspecific urethritis caused by, **2:**67
pneumonia caused by, **2:**73
Proximity
body language and, **5:**19
friendship and, **5:**46–47
Psilocybin, **7:**61
Psoriasis, **1:**69, **2:**76, **3:**98–99
Psychedelics. *See* Hallucinogens
Psychiatric social workers, **9:**36
Psychiatrists, **5:**75, 76, **9:**34, 36
Psychiatry, **5:**75. *See also* Drug therapy, **5:**39–40; Electroconvulsive therapy (ECT), **5:**41; Psychotherapy, **5:**79–82
Psychoactive drugs, **7:**51, 52, 84–85
cocaine as, **7:**38
dangers of abuse of, **7:**85
hallucinogens, **7:**60–61
narcotic analgesics, **7:**16
types of, **7:**84
See also Psychotherapy, **5:**79–82; Addiction, **7:**4–5; Alcoholism, **7:**12–14; Antidepressants, **7:**23–24; Barbiturates, **7:**31–32; Drug use and abuse, **7:**55–57; Inhalants, **7:**65–66; Marijuana, **7:**71–73; Narcotics, **7:**76–78; Sedatives, **7:**87–88; Stimulants, **7:**95–96
Psychoanalysis, **5:**75, 76, 79–80
Psychoanalysts, **9:**36
Psychoanalytic theories of personality, **5:**69
Psychodynamic therapy, **5:**79–80
Psychogenic amnesia, **5:**7
Psychological cravings, **4:**55, *55*
Psychological dependence, **7:**4, 73
on alcohol, **7:**8
on sedatives, **7:**88
Psychologically based psychotherapy, **5:**79–81
Psychologist, **5:**75, 76, **9:**36
Psychology, **5:**76–78
developmental, **5:**34–36
fields of, **5:**77–78
health, **5:**44, 49
history of, **5:**76–77
See also Psychotherapists, **9:**35–36
Psychopath. *See* Antisocial personality
Psychopharmacologists, **5:**77. *See also* Drug therapy, **5:**39–40
Psychosis (psychotic disorder), **5:**39, 60, 78. *See also* Depression, **5:**32–34; Drug therapy, **5:**39–40; Mental illness, **5:**60–61; Neurosis, **5:**65; Schizophrenia, **5:**86

Psychosomatic disorders, 5:44, 78–79. *See also* Hysteria, 5:53
Psychosurgery, 5:82
Psychotherapists, 9:35–36. *See also* Psychiatry, 5:75; Psychology, 5:76–78; Psychotherapy, 5:79–82
Psychotherapy, 5:79–82
    aims of, 9:35–36
    biologically based, 5:79, 81–82
    drug therapy and, 5:39–40
    group, 5:81
    for hyperactivity, 5:51
    for mental illness, 5:61
    for multiple personality, 5:65
    psychologically based, 5:79–81
    for schizophrenia, 5:39, 86
Puberty, 1:5, 43, 79, 82, 6:79–80
    acne and, 3:4
    male reproductive system at, 6:52
    menarche and, 6:59, 79
    nocturnal emission during, 6:54, 67, 80
    physical changes in, 6:79–80
    sex hormones activated in, 6:84
    sexual attraction and, 6:87
    social and emotional changes in, 6:80
    See also Adolescence, 1:5–6; Pregnancy, 6:74–76; Sexuality, 6:92; Teenage pregnancy, 6:97–98
Pubic lice, 2:57
Pubic symphysis, 1:77
Pubis, 1:77
Public health, 9:34–35
    drugs and, 7:53–54
Public Health Service, 9:8–10
Public sanitation efforts, 8:80
Public transportation, use of, 8:34
Public water conservation methods, 8:94–95
Puerperal sepsis, 2:74
Pulmonary artery, 1:12, 26, 48
Pulmonary circulation, 1:26
Pulmonary embolism, 3:86
Pulmonary fibrosis, 3:86
Pulmonary vein, 1:26, 84, 102
Pulp, tooth, 1:99
Pulse, 1:26, 8:72, 72
    normal, 8:57
    taking a, 4:68
    See also Circulatory system, 1:25–27; Bleeding, 8:18–19
Puncture wound, 8:101
Punishment, 5:56
    behavior modification using, 5:17
    caution in using, 5:27
    operant conditioning using, 5:26, 27

Pupil, 1:39, 40
Purchasing food, 4:63
Pure Food and Drug Act (1906), 7:53
Pus, 2:74–75
    abscess and, 2:4
    in boil, 2:16
    conjunctivitis and, 2:26
    inflammation and, 2:51
    See also Infection, 2:50–51
Pustules, 3:4, *4*
Pyridoxine (B₆), 4:*116*, 117, *121*

Quaalude. *See* Sedatives
Quackery, 9:37–38. *See also* Fad diets, 4:42–43; Placebo, 7:81–82
Quadrantectomy, 6:56
Quadriceps muscles, 1:58
Quadriplegia, 3:95
Quadruplets, 6:62
Quick breads, 4:17
Quinine, 2:60
Quinlan, Karen Ann, 9:21
Quintuplets, 6:62
Quitting smoking, 7:85–87, 91
    difficulty of, 7:85–86
    health benefits of, 7:85
    methods of, 7:83, 86–87
    See also Tobacco, 7:97–99

Rabies, 2:75, 8:16, 55
Racism, 5:73
Radial artery, taking pulse in, 8:72
Radial keratotomy, 3:117
Radiation, 8:72–74
    ionizing, 8:72, 73
    limiting exposure to, 8:73–74
    nonionizing, 8:72, 73
    ozone layer and protection from, 8:10, 64
    prenatal, 6:12
    from radioactive waste, 8:48–49, 62, 73
    from radon, 8:73, 74
    solar, 8:83
    ultraviolet (UV), 8:10, 64, 65, 73, 74, 88–89
    See also Cancer, 3:29–32; Magnetic resonance imaging, 3:88; Skin cancer, 3:102–3; X-ray examination, 3:117–18; Hazardous waste, 8:47–49; Sun damage, 8:88–89
Radiation sickness, 8:62
Radiation therapy, 3:31, 99, 7:22. *See also* Cancer, 3:29–32

Radical hysterectomy, 6:48
Radical mastectomy, 3:27, 6:57
Radioactive iodine uptake (RAIU) test, 3:112
Radioactive waste, 8:48–49, 62, 73
Radiologic technologists, 9:23
Radiologist, 9:34, 38–39. *See also* Magnetic resonance imaging, 3:88; Radiation therapy, 3:99; X-ray examination, 3:117–18; Ultrasound, 6:100; Radiation, 8:72–74
Radiology departments, 9:20
Radius, 1:34
Radon, 8:74
    air pollution caused by, 8:9
    ionizing radiation from, 8:73, 74
    See also Lung cancer, 3:85
Rahe, Richard, 5:4, 96
Ramps, access, 8:4–5
Rape, 6:80–82, 92, 8:92
    common misconceptions about, 6:80–81
    date, 6:27–28
    getting help after, 6:81–82
    risk factors for, 6:80, 81, *81*
    See also Violence, 8:92–93
Rapid eye movement (REM), 1:92, 5:37–38
Rash, 2:76–77
    of allergies, 3:6
    causes of, 2:76
    of chicken pox, 2:19
    contact poisoning and, 8:70
    of eczema, 3:51
    of lupus, 3:87
    of measles, 2:61
    of psoriasis, 3:98–99
    of scarlet fever, 2:81
    seborrheic dermatitis, 3:43
    of shingles, 2:83
    See also Skin, 1:89–90; Fungal infections, 2:38–39; Itching, 2:54; Meningitis, 2:61–62; Parasitic infections, 2:68–69; Rubella, 2:78–79
RAST (radioallergosorbent test), 3:8, 9
Rationalization, 5:32
Raynaud's disease, 3:100
Raynaud's phenomenon, 3:100. *See also* Arteriosclerosis, 3:15; Arthritis, 3:15–17; Blood clot, 3:24
Reaction formation, 5:32
Reading disorders, 5:58
Reading machines, 8:4
Rebound, 7:27
Receptors, 1:52, 71, 5:68
Receptor theory, 7:80–81
Recessive gene, 3:42, 91, 6:41

Recessive inheritance, 6:41–42

Recombinant DNA, 8:44

Recommended dietary allowance (RDA), 4:92–93
  on food labels, 4:56, *92*, 93
  of minerals, 4:*80*
  of vitamins, 4:*121*, 122
  See also Dietary guidelines, 4:28–29

Reconstructive surgery. *See* Plastic surgery

Recovery programs for alcoholics, 7:14

Recovery stage of infection, 2:51

Recreation, safety equipment for, 8:79

Recreational drugs, 7:6, 52
  alcohol, 7:6–9
  cocaine, 7:37–38
  marijuana, 7:71–73
  tobacco, 7:97–99

Rectal infections, chlamydial, 2:21

Rectal thermometer, 8:19

Rectum, 1:10–11, 81, *81*
  colorectal cancer in, 3:40
  hemorrhoids in lining of, 3:75, *75*
  See also Digestive system, 1:30–33

Recuperation, 4:94

Recycling, 8:74–76
  reducing solid waste by, 8:85–86

Red blood cells (erythrocytes), 1:12–13, 18, 22, 100, 3:11, 12, 102, *102*

Reference books, self-care, 8:57

Referred pain, 3:94

Reflex
  knee-jerk, 1:81
  vomiting, 2:98

Reflex action, 1:72–73, 81–82, 92. *See also* Hypothalamus, 1:52

Reflex arc, 1:72–73, 81

Refrigeration, 4:59

Registered dietitian (RD), 9:26

Registered nurse (R.N.), 9:24

Regression, 5:32

Rehabilitation
  drug, 7:49–50
  after stroke, 3:108

Rehabilitation center, 9:39–40. *See also* Psychotherapy, 5:79–82; Drug rehabilitation, 7:49–50; Nursing home, 9:25; Occupational therapist, 9:26–27; Physical therapist, 9:30–31; Speech therapy, 9:40–41

Reinforcement, 5:17, 26, 56

Reiter's syndrome, 2:67

Rejection of transplant, 3:73, 113

Relationships, 5:82–83
  codependency, 7:39–40
  conflict resolution and, 5:27–28
  coping and positive, 5:29–30
  dating, 6:28–29
  family, 5:44–45
  friendships, 5:46–47, 83
  happiness and, 5:48
  harmful, 5:83
  impact of, 5:82–83
  intimacy and, 5:54
  love, 5:58–59
  shyness and, 5:91
  social skills and, 5:94–95
  stages of, 5:83

Relaxation, 4:93–94

Relaxation response, 5:84

Relaxation training, 5:84
  biofeedback, 5:18, 84, 99
  for natural childbirth, 6:64
  stress management through, 5:30, 84, 97, 98–99

Releasing factors, 1:52

REM (rapid eye movement) sleep, 1:92, 5:37–38

Renal failure. *See* Kidney failure

Repression, 5:31

Reproduction, cell, 1:23

Reproductive cells, 1:23

Reproductive systems, 1:82–84
  female, 6:33–34
  male, 6:52–54
  menstruation and, 6:59–61
  steroid use and risk to, 7:94–95

Rescue squads, 8:32

Research, medical, 9:22

Reservatrol, 4:89

Reservoirs, 2:51, 8:94

Residency, 9:32

Residential-care facilities (RCFs), 9:25

Resistance equipment, 4:42

Resistance stage of general adaptation syndrome, 5:96, 97

Resistance to antibiotics, 7:21–22

Resolution stage of sexual response cycle, 6:93

Respiratory distress syndrome, 6:77

Respiratory infections, *Chlamydia trachomatis* and, 2:21

Respiratory problems, smoking and, 1:85–86, 7:91

Respiratory system, 1:84–86, *85*
  air pollution's effect on, 8:9
  and diaphragm, 1:30
  lungs, 1:62–63
  nose, 1:75–76
  See also Circulatory system, 1:25–27; Mouth, 1:65–66;

Common cold, 2:23–24; Asthma, 3:17–19

Respondent conditioning. *See* Classical conditioning

Responsibility, 5:84–85
  diffusion of, 5:74

Rest, 4:93–94
  relaxation training and, 5:84
  sleep and, 1:91–92
  sleep problems and, 5:93–94
  See also Energy, physical, 4:36–38; Fatigue, 4:44–45; Lifestyle, 4:71–72; Stress-management techniques, 5:98–99

Resting heart rate, 4:68

Restraining orders, 8:86

Restrictive breathing disorder, 2:17

Retainer, 3:92

Retardation. *See* Mental retardation

Retina, 1:40, *40*
  detached, 3:55, *55*

Retin-A, 7:19

Retinol. *See* Vitamin A

Retirement, 1:8

Retrovirus, HIV, 2:5, 45–46

Rewards, behavior modification using, 5:17

Reye's syndrome, 2:20, 38, 53, 3:100
  aspirin and, 2:20, 38, 53, 7:30
  See also Coma, 3:40–41

Rheumatic fever, 2:77–78. *See also* Heart, 1:47–49; Bacterial infections, 2:13–15; Culture, 2:28–29; Inflammation, 2:51–52; Streptococcal infections, 2:86–87; Tonsillitis, 2:91–92; Heart disease, 3:69–72

Rheumatoid arthritis, 1:28, 50, 56, 59, 69, 88, 3:16–17

Rheumatoid nodules, 3:16

Rh factor, 1:14, 17, 6:82. *See also* Blood, 1:12–14; Blood type, 1:17; Blood transfusion, 3:25; Genetics, 6:40–42

Rhinoplasty, 3:97

Rib cage, 1:23

Rib injury, 1:24

Riboflavin, 4:*116*, 117, *121*

Rice, 4:17

RICE (rest, ice, compression, and elevation), 1:10, 56, 4:102, 8:76–77, *76*, 87. *See also* Sports injuries, 4:102–5; First aid, 8:38–39

Rickets, 1:18, 4:19, 119

Rickettsias, 2:64, 78, 96

RID (Remove Intoxicated Drivers), 7:47

Rights
  nonsmokers', 8:60–61
  patients', 9:29

Right-to-die laws, 9:21

Ringworm, 1:90, 2:39

Risk factors, 4:94–95. *See also* Heredity and environment, 5:49–50

Ritalin, 5:51, 7:87. *See also* Hyperactivity, 5:50–51

Rites of passage, 6:80

RNA. *See* Genetics

Rocky Mountain spotted fever, 2:78

Rodents
diseases spread by, 2:71, 72, 96
food contamination by, 4:62

Rods, 1:40

Roe v. Wade, 6:5

Rogers, Carl, 5:77, 80

Role confusion, identity versus, 5:35

Role model, 5:85. *See also* Adult identity, 5:4–5; Developmental psychology, 5:34–36; Family, 5:44–45; Heredity and environment, 5:49–50; Self-image, 5:89–90; Social skills, 5:94–95

Roles
gender, 5:90
sex, 6:85–86

Romantic love, 5:36, 59

Root canal treatment, 3:45

Root of tooth, 1:99

Rotaviruses, 2:97

Roughage. *See* Fiber

Rowing machines, 4:41

Rubber. *See* Condom

Rubella, 2:61, 78–79, 3:35, 36, 67, 72
MMR vaccine for, 2:61, 66, 79
during pregnancy, 2:61, 78, 79, 3:35, 36, 67, 72, 6:12, 75
See also Scarlet fever, 2:81–82

Rubeola. *See* Measles

Runner's knee, 1:59

Running, 4:24, 95–96. *See also* Aerobic exercise, 4:4–6; Body composition, 4:13–14; Endurance, 4:34–35; Fitness, 4:48–49; Heart rate, 4:68; Sports injuries, 4:102–5

Sabin oral vaccine, 2:74

Saccharin, 4:8–9

Sacroiliac joints, 1:77

Sacrum, 1:77, *94*

Sadism, 6:9

Sadness. *See* Emotion

Safer sex, 6:82–83, 91
masturbation and, 6:57, 83
preventing HIV infection with, 2:7–8, 46
prevention of STDs with, 6:82–83, 95

See also AIDS, 2:4–8; Anal sex, 6:8; Contraception, 6:24–26; Sexual intercourse, 6:91–92

Safety
automobile, 8:11–13
cycling, 4:25–26, 8:14
drinking and driving and, 7:47, 8:12
electrical, 8:30–31
fire, 8:36–37
food, 4:58, 61–63
home, 8:51–53
running, 4:96
water, 8:98–99
weight training, 4:133
See also Safety on the job, 8:79–80

Safety equipment, 8:77–79
electrical, 8:30–31
in home, 8:77–78
for recreation, 8:79
in vehicle, 8:78
in workplace, 8:78, 80
See also Hearing loss, 3:66–67; Accidents, 8:5–6; Automobile safety, 8:11–13; Bicycle safety, 8:14; Fire safety, 8:36–37; Injuries, 8:55–56; Noise pollution, 8:59–60; Water safety, 8:98–99

Safety on the job, 8:79–80
accidents in workplace, 8:5, 59, 79
equipment for, 8:78, 80
noise pollution and, 8:59
OSHA and, 8:62–63
See also Particulates, 8:65–66

Salicylic acid, 7:30

Saline laxatives, 7:69

Saliva, 1:32, 65, 86
HIV transmission through, 2:8, 46

Salivary glands, 1:65, 86, *86*
mumps and swelling of, 2:66

Salk vaccine, 2:74

Salmonella food poisoning, 2:80, 4:57, 62

Salmonella infections, 2:80. *See also* Bacterial infections, 2:13–15; Typhoid fever, 2:96

Salmonella typhosa, 2:96

Salt, 4:96–97, 98
low-sodium (low-salt) diet, 4:31, 98–99
as preservative, 4:52
See also Hypertension, 3:77–78; Minerals, 4:79–81; Monosodium glutamate (MSG), 4:82; Potassium, 4:89

Sanitary pads, 6:34, 35, 60

Sanitation, 8:80–81
antiseptics for, 7:28–29
See also Communicable disease, 2:24–26; Infection, 2:50–51; Home safety, 8:51–53; Water pollution, 8:95–97

Sarcoidosis, 1:86

Sarcoma, 3:30, 81–82
Kaposi's, 2:5, 6, 3:81–82

Sarcoptes scabiei, 2:81

Satiety, 4:8

Saturated fats, 4:24, *24*, 45, 46, 47, 77

Scabies, 2:81

Scaling, 3:51, 98

Scalp, dandruff and, 3:43

Scalp ringworm, treating, 7:25

Scapegoat theory of prejudice, 5:73

Scapula, 1:87–88

Scarlet fever, 2:81–82. *See also* Rheumatic fever, 2:77–78; Sore throat, 2:85–86; Streptococcal infections, 2:86–87; Tonsillitis, 2:91–92

Scarring, 1:86–87
of multiple sclerosis, 3:*90*

Schachter-Singer theory of emotion, 5:43, *43*

Schizoid personality disorder, 5:70

Schizophrenia, 5:86
drug therapy for, 5:39, 86
hallucinations of, 5:48, 86
paranoid, 5:67
See also Psychosis (psychotic disorder), 5:78

Schizotypal personality disorder, 5:67, 70

Schlemm, canal of, 3:60, *60*

School, sex roles reinforced in, 6:86

School psychology, 5:77

Sciatica, 3:21

Sclera, 1:39

Scoliosis, 1:94, 3:100–101

Scorpion stings, 8:17

Screening
of donated blood, 3:25, 75
genetic, 6:42–44

Screening mammograms, 6:54, 55

Scrotum, 1:83, 6:52

Scrub typhus, 2:96

Scurvy, 4:73, 117

Sea anemones, stings from, 8:17–18

Sea creatures, stings from, 8:17–18

Sealant, dental, 3:45

Seasonal affective disorder (SAD), 5:34

Seat belts, 8:11–12, *11*, 78

Sea urchins, stings from, 8:18

Sebaceous glands, 1:45, 89, 3:4, *4*

Seborrheic dermatitis, 3:43
Sebum, 3:4
Secobarbital, 7:17
Second Amendment of the Constitution, 8:47
Secondary emotion, 5:43
Secondary hypertension, 3:78
Secondary infections, 7:21
Secondary sex characteristics, 6:84–85
Secondary tumor, 3:25
Second-degree burns, 8:20, *20*
Secondhand smoke, 3:85, 7:92, 8:60
Sedatives, 7:51, 84, 87–88, *88*
 barbiturates, 7:31–32
 sleeping pills, 7:90
 See also Alcohol, 7:6–9; Drug interaction, 7:47–48; Drug overdose, 7:48–49; Drug rehabilitation, 7:49–50; Drug use and abuse, 7:55–57; Psychoactive drugs, 7:84–85
Sedimentation, 8:97
Seizure disorder. *See* Epilepsy
Selegiline (Deprenyl or Eldepryl), 3:96
Selenium, 4:*80*, 81
Self-actualization, 5:70, 87. *See also* Psychology, 5:76–78; Psychotherapy, 5:79–82
Self-care, medical, 8:56–57
Self-concept. *See* Self-image
Self-efficacy, 5:88. *See also* Assertiveness, 5:12–13; Coping skills, 5:29–30; Self-actualization, 5:87; Self-image, 5:89–90
Self-esteem, 5:70, 88–89
 developing and building, 5:89
 happiness and, 5:48
 sex roles and, 6:85
 See also Assertiveness, 5:12–13; Psychotherapy, 5:79–82; Self-actualization, 5:87; Self-efficacy, 5:88
Self-help groups, 7:5, 14, 50
Self-image, 5:89–90
 gender identity and, 6:39
 incest and, 6:49
 self-actualization and, 5:87
 self-efficacy and, 5:88
 sex roles and, 6:85
 See also Role model, 5:85
Selye, Hans, 5:96
Semen, 1:83, 6:53, 84
 fertilization by, 6:35–37
 HIV transmission through, 2:5, 46
 nocturnal emission of, 6:54, 67, 80

 See also Infertility, 6:50–51; Male reproductive system, 6:52–54; Sexual intercourse, 6:91–92
Semicircular canals, 1:33, 34
Seminal fluid, 6:84
Seminal vesicles, 1:83, 6:53
Semivegetarians, 4:113
Senile dementia, 5:90
Senility, 3:9, 5:90–91. *See also* Alzheimer's disease, 3:9–10; Dementia, 3:43–44; Stroke, 3:106–8; Anxiety, 5:9–10; Depression, 5:32–34; Organic brain disorders, 5:66
Sensorimotor stage, 5:35
Sensorineural deafness, 3:67
Sensory deafness, 8:59
Sensory nerves, 3:94
Sensory neurons, 1:71–72, 74, 81, 93
Septicemia, 2:14
Septic shock, 3:25, 101
Septic tanks, 8:82
Septum, 1:47, 75
 deviated, 1:76, 89
Serum, blood, 1:13
 antiserum made of, 2:11–12
 gamma globulin, 2:39
Set-point theory of weight, 4:16
Sewage, 8:81–82
 disposal problems, 8:82
 sanitation and, 8:80–81
 treatment processes, 8:82
 waste management and, 8:93–94
 water purity and, 8:94–95, 97–98
Sex
 anal, 2:7–8, 46, 6:8, 94
 oral, 6:67, 94
 See also Sexual intercourse, 6:91–92
Sex change operation, 6:99
Sex determination, 6:40
Sex hormones, 1:5–6, 7, 6:84–85
 breast changes due to, 6:13
 breast-feeding preparation and, 6:14
 hormonal change during menopause, 6:58
 ovulation and, 6:68
 production of, 6:33, 52, 72
 sexual attraction and, 6:87
 See also Female reproductive system, 6:33–34; Male reproductive system, 6:52–54
Sexism, 5:73
Sex-linked inheritance, 6:42
Sex organs, male and female, 6:*18*
 cancers of, 6:17–18
 See also Female reproductive system, 6:33–34; Male reproductive system, 6:52–54

Sex roles, 6:39, 85–86. *See also* Gender identity, 6:38–40
Sex therapy, 6:89
Sexual abuse, 6:87, 8:23
 date rape, 6:27–28
 incest, 6:49–50
 rape, 6:80–82, 92
 See also Pornography, 6:72–73; Child abuse, 8:22–23; Spouse abuse, 8:86; Violence, 8:92–93
Sexual arousal, 6:33, 93
Sexual attraction, 6:87–88
 bisexuality, 6:12–13
 dating and, 6:28–29
 heterosexuality, 6:45–46
 homosexuality, 6:46–-48
Sexual behavior
 atypical, 6:9
 in marriage, 6:55–56
 masturbation, 6:57–58
 after menopause, 6:58–59
 safer sex, 6:57, 82–83, 91, 95
Sexual characteristics, 1:5
Sexual dysfunction, 6:88–89, 91. *See also* Psychotherapists, 9:35–36
Sexual fantasies, 6:89–90. *See also* Intimacy, 5:54; Sexual attraction, 6:87–88
Sexual intercourse, 6:91–92
 abstinence from, 6:5, 24, 83, 95
 anal sex, 2:7–8, 46, 6:8, 94
 contraception use in, 6:24–26
 date rape, 6:27–28
 individual differences and, 6:91
 natural family planning and, 6:5, 24, 25, 66
 oral sex and, 6:67
 orgasm and, 6:54, 67–68, 91, 93
 personal decision and, 6:92
 physical aspects of, 6:91
 responsibility and, 6:91
 See also AIDS, 2:4–8
Sexuality, 6:92
 bisexuality, 6:12–13
 heterosexuality, 6:45–46
 homosexuality, 6:46–48
Sexually transmitted diseases (STDs), 2:82, 6:94–95, *94*
 AIDS, 2:4–8
 chlamydial infections, 2:20–21
 genital herpes, 2:44
 gonorrhea, 2:41–42
 HIV, 2:45–46
 infertility caused by, 6:51
 nonspecific urethritis, 2:67
 pelvic inflammatory disease after, 2:70

prevention of spread of, 6:22–23, 26, 82–83, 95
safer sex and, 6:82–83
spread of, 6:8, 94–95
syphilis, 2:87–88
treatment for, 6:95
See also Bacterial infections, 2:13–15; Genital warts, 2:40; Herpes infections, 2:44–45; Viral infections, 2:97–98
Sexual materials, pornographic, 6:72–73
Sexual orientation, 1:6. *See also* Sexuality, 6:92
Sexual response cycle, 6:91, 92–93. *See also* Female reproductive system, 6:33–34; Male reproductive system, 6:52–54; Sexuality, 6:92
Shame and doubt, autonomy versus, 5:35
Shampoo, dandruff, 7:41
Shellfish, 4:76
Shell shock. *See* Post-traumatic stress disorder (PTSD)
Shingles, 2:83–84, 3:91. *See also* Immune system, 1:52–55; Chicken pox, 2:19–20
Shinsplints, 4:*103*, 104
Shivering, 1:73
Shock, 3:14, 101, *101*
anaphylactic, 3:6, 79, 101, 4:53, 7:21, 25, 47, 8:17
burns and, 8:20
electric, 8:31, *31*
internal bleeding and, 8:18
septic, 3:25, 101
symptoms of, 8:18
thermal, 8:91
toxic shock syndrome, 2:92–93
treating, 8:*38*, 39
See also Bleeding, 8:18–19; First aid, 8:38–39
Shoulder, 1:87–88, 87
dislocated, 8:*26*
See also Bursitis, 3:28
Shyness, 5:91. *See also* Social skills, 5:94–95
Siamese twins, 6:62
Sibling rivalry, 5:83, 92
Sickle cell anemia, 1:23, 3:12, 102, *102*, 6:42. *See also* Birth defects, 6:11–12; Genetic screening, 6:42–44; Genetic counselor, 9:12
Side effects, 7:89
of amphetamines, 7:15
of anabolic steroids, 7:94–95
of antacids, 7:18–19
of antibiotics, 7:21
of anticancer drugs, 7:22

of antidepressants, 7:24
of antidiarrheal products, 7:24
of antifungal agents, 7:25
of antihistamines and decongestants, 7:26, *26*
of antihypertensives, 7:27
of antiviral drugs, 7:30
of aspirin, 7:30
of AZT, 7:31
of barbiturates, 7:32
of beta-blockers, 7:32
of bronchodilators, 7:34
of caffeine, 7:35–36
of corticosteroids, 7:40
of diet pills, 7:44
drug interactions and, 7:45–46, 48
of general anesthetics, 7:17
handling, 7:89
of hormone replacement therapy, 7:63
of L-dopa, 7:70
of methadone, 7:74
of nonprescription drugs, 7:79, 89
of penicillin, 7:80
from placebos, 7:82
of ritalin, 7:87
of sedatives, 7:88
of sleeping pills, 7:90
of sulfa drugs, 7:97
types of, 7:89
See also Drug allergy, 7:47; Drug interaction, 7:47–48; Drug use and abuse, 7:55–57; Prescription drugs, 7:82–83
Sideroblastic anemia, 3:12
Sidestream smoke, 7:92, 8:60
Sierra Club, 8:35
Sigmoidoscopy, 3:39
Silicone-gel breast implants, 6:15
Similarities, friendship and, 5:46–47
Simple carbohydrates, 4:21, 22, 106
Simple fracture, 8:41
Simple mastectomy, 3:27, 6:57
Single-parent family, 5:44–45
Single parenthood, 6:70
Sinus(es), 1:84, 88–89, *88*
Sinusitis, 1:89, 2:84–85, *84*. *See also* Antihistamines and decongestants, 7:25–27
Situational shyness, 5:91
Situational use, addiction and, 7:5
Skeletal muscles, 1:67, 68
Skeleton, 1:17–18, 68, *68*, 69
Skilled-care nursing homes, 9:39
Skilled nursing facilities (SNFs), 9:25
Ski machine, 4:41

Skin, 1:46, 89–90, *90*
acne and, 3:4–5
blisters on, 3:23–24
dandruff, 3:43
dry, itching due to, 2:54
eczema and, 3:51
impetigo, 2:49–50
psoriasis and, 3:98–99
rashes on, 2:76–77
scarring on, 1:86–87
sunscreens for, 1:90, 7:97, 8:89
warts on, 2:99–100
yellow, jaundice and, 3:81
See also Immune system, 1:52–55; Nails, 1:69
Skin allergy. *See* Contact dermatitis
Skin biopsy, 3:23
Skin cancer, 1:90, 3:102–3
sun damage and, 3:102, 103, 8:88–89
ultraviolet radiation and, 8:65, 73
See also Kaposi's sarcoma, 3:81–82
Skin cells, 1:22
Skin grafts, 3:97
Skinner, B. F., 5:26, 77
Skin test, 3:8–9
Skull, 1:*68*, 69, 91. *See also* Musculoskeletal system, 1:68–69
Sleep, 1:91–92, 4:93
dreams during, 5:37–39
REM (rapid eye movement), 1:92, 5:37–38
Sleep apnea, 1:92, 3:103, 104
Sleep disorders, 3:56, 103–4
Sleeping pills, 7:90. *See also* Antihistamines and decongestants, 7:25–27
Sleep problems, 5:93–94
circadian rhythms and, 5:22
relaxation training for, 5:84
stress-management techniques for, 5:98–99
Sleepwalking, 5:94
Slim disease, 2:5. *See also* AIDS, 2:4–8
Slipped disk, 1:94, 3:21–22
Slow viruses, 2:97
Slow-wave sleep, 1:91, *92*
Small intestine, 1:32
hookworms in, 2:69
Smallpox, 2:85. *See also* Epidemic, 2:36
Smell, sense of, 1:75
Smog, 8:82
air pollution and, 8:9, 82
ozone in, 8:64, 90
temperature inversion and, 8:90

toxic substances in, 8:91
See also Acid rain, 8:6–7; Particulates, 8:65–66
Smoke detectors, 8:52, 77
Smoke inhalation, 8:83. *See also*
Shock, 3:101; Burns, 8:20–21; Fire safety, 8:36–37; First aid, 8:38–39; Toxic substances, 8:91–92
Smoking, 6:12, 7:90–92
addiction to, 7:85–86
dangers of, 8:60
fire safety and, 8:37
hazards of, 1:85–86, 3:19, *20*, 32, 53, *71,* 7:90–91
laws about, 7:98–99, 8:60–61
lung cancer and, 2:36–37, 3:85
nonsmokers' rights and, 8:60–61
passive, 8:60
quitting, 7:83, 85–87, 91
reasons for, 7:92
secondhand smoke, 7:92
surgeon general on, 7:98–99
See also Cardiovascular disease, 3:34; Addiction, 7:4–5; Chewing tobacco and snuff, 7:36; Tobacco, 7:97–99
Smooth muscles, 1:67
Snack food, 4:97. *See also* Fast food, 4:43; Junk food, 4:70–71; Weight management, 4:130–32
Snake bites, 8:17
Snappers, 7:66
Snellen chart, 3:55, *55*
Snoring, 1:5
Snowstorms, 8:101
Snuff, 7:36
Social age, 9:13
Social development, 5:35–36
Social drinking, 7:92–93
alcoholism development and, 7:12, 93
See also Drinking and driving, 7:46–47
Social health, 5:60
Socialized medicine, 9:14
Social psychiatry, 5:75
Social psychology, 5:77
Social Readjustment Rating Scale, 5:96
Social Security Administration, 9:8
Social skills, 5:94–95
communication, 5:22–23
conflict resolution and, 5:27–28
friendship and, 5:46–47
shyness and, 5:91
Social worker
hospital, 9:18
psychiatric, 9:36
Society, values of, 5:100–101

Sociopath. *See* Antisocial personality
Sodium, 4:79, *80,* 89, 97–99
in urine, 1:57
See also Hypertension, 3:77–78; Calcium, 4:19–20; Potassium, 4:89; Vitamins, 4:121–22; Water, 4:123–24
Sodium bicarbonate (baking soda), 4:98
Sodium chloride. *See* Salt
Sodium pentothal, 7:17
Sodium propionate, 4:52
Soft drinks, 4:11
Solar batteries, 8:84
Solar energy, 8:83–84
Solar furnaces, 8:84
Solar plexus, 1:4
Solid waste, 8:84–86. *See also* Sanitation, 8:80–81
Soluble fiber, 4:47
Soluble proteins, 4:91
Solvents, 7:66
Somatic nervous system, 1:73
Somatoform disorders, 5:78–79
Sonography. *See* Ultrasound
Sore muscles, 4:104
Sore throat, 1:96, 2:85–86
of tonsillitis, 2:91–92
See also Throat, 1:95–96; Antibiotic treatment, 2:8–10; Chicken pox, 2:19–20; Common cold, 2:23–24; Influenza, 2:52–53; Mononucleosis, 2:65; Rheumatic fever, 2:77–78; Scarlet fever, 2:81–82; Streptococcal infections, 2:86–87
Spastic cerebral palsy, 3:37
Special education programs, 5:58
Specialists, 9:33–34
in surgery, 9:41
Speculum, 6:45, *69*
Speech, 5:22
Speech disorders, 3:104–5
access for people with, 8:4
speech therapy for, 9:40–41
Speech-language pathologists, 9:40–41
Speech therapy, 3:37, 104–5, 9:40–41. *See also* Speech disorders, 3:104–5
Speed. *See* Amphetamines
Sperm, 1:82
fertilization process and, 6:35–36
production of, 6:52–53
in semen, 6:84
Sperm count, 6:51
Spermicides, 6:24, *25,* 93–94
contraceptive devices using, 6:18, 23, 29
safer sex using, 2:7, 46

Sphenoid sinuses, 1:88
Sphincter muscles, 1:10
Sphygmomanometer, 1:15, 3:78
Spider bites, 8:17
Spinal cord, 1:70, 93–94, *93,* 5:20. *See also* Nervous system, 1:71–74; Neuron, 1:74–75; Reflex action, 1:81–82
Spinal fracture, 8:42
Spinal meninges, 1:93
Spinal tap. *See* Lumbar puncture
Spine, 1:94–95, *94*
scoliosis of, 3:100–101
See also Musculoskeletal system, 1:68–69; Back problems, 3:21–22
Spirilla or spirochetes, 2:13, *15,* 63, 88
Spiritual health, 5:60
Spleen, hemolytic anemia and, 3:12
Splinters, removing, 8:56
Splinting, 8:42
Spontaneous abortion. *See* Miscarriage
Sports
abuse of drugs in, 7:52–53
safety equipment for, 8:79
Sports and fitness, 4:99–101, *99*
athletic footwear for, 4:9–10
calories burned in various activities, 4:36
choosing a sport, 4:99–100
fitness training, 4:49–50
President's Council on Physical Fitness and Sports, 4:90
training for sports, 4:100–101
See also Endurance, 4:34–35; Flexibility, 4:51–52; Sports injuries, 4:102–5; Strength, 4:107
Sports and heat problems, 4:101–2
heatstroke, 8:49–50, 99
See also Dehydration, 4:26–27; Exercise, 4:39–40; Perspiration, 4:87–88
Sports injuries, 1:28, 35, 59, 4:25, 102–5, *103*
common types of, 4:102–4
treating and preventing, 4:104–5, 106
See also Pain, 3:94; Athletic footwear, 4:9–10; Strength exercise, 4:108–9; Stretching exercise, 4:109–10; First aid, 8:38–39
Sports medicine, 4:105–6. *See also* Physical therapist, 9:30–31; Physicians (M.D.'s), 9:31–34; Podiatrist, 9:34
Sports medicine centers, 9:39

Sports psychologists, 4:106
Spouse abuse, 8:86, 92, 93. *See also* Child abuse, 8:22–23; Violence, 8:92–93
Sprains and strains, 8:55–56, 86–88, 87
　first aid for, 8:55–56, 87
　preventing, 8:87–88
　sports and, 4:*103*, 104
　See also Ankle, 1:9–10; Connective tissue, 1:27–28; Knee, 1:58–59; Muscles, 1:66–67; Analgesics, 7:15–17; Dislocations, 8:26; RICE (rest, ice, compression, and elevation), 8:76–77
Sprue, nontropical, 4:32
Squamous cell carcinoma, 3:102
Stagnation, generativity versus, 5:36
Stamina. *See* Endurance
Stapes (stirrup), 1:33, 34
Staphylococci, 2:13, 14
　infection by, 2:15–16, 68
Staphylococcus aureus, 2:93
　food poisoning caused by, 4:57
Starch, 4:21, 106–7
　in breads and cereals group, 4:17–18
　See also Carbohydrates, 4:21–22; Energy, food, 4:35–36; Nutrients, 4:82–84
Static stretching, 4:109, *109*
Stationary bicycles, 4:40–41
STDs. *See* Sexually transmitted diseases (STDs)
Stepparents, 6:70
Stereotypes, 5:13, 72–73
　sex-role, 6:85–86
Sterilization, 4:59, 6:25, 96–97, *96*
　hysterectomy, 6:48–49
　See also Female reproductive system, 6:33–34; Male reproductive system, 6:52–54
Sternum, 1:23, 24, *24*, 87
Steroids, 7:94–95
　for allergies, 3:7
　anabolic, 4:13, 7:94–95
　hormone therapy using, 7:64
　side effects and risks of, 7:94–95
　uses and abuses of, 7:52–53, 94
　See also Corticosteroids, 7:40; Drug use and abuse, 7:55–57
Stiff neck, 1:70
Stillbirth, 6:61
Still's disease, 3:17
Stimulant laxatives, 7:69
Stimulants, 4:27, 7:51, 84, 95–96
　abused by athletes, 7:52
　amphetamines, 7:15

antidepressants, 7:23–24
caffeine, 7:35–36
cocaine, 7:37–38
effects of, 7:95
ritalin, 7:87
smoking, 7:90–92
types of, 7:96
See also Drug use and abuse, 7:55–57; Psychoactive drugs, 7:84–85
Stings. *See* Bites and stings
Stirrup (stapes), 1:*33*, 34
Stomach, 1:31
　vomiting of contents of, 2:98–99
Stomachache/indigestion, 3:105–6. *See also* Abdomen, 1:4; Digestive system, 1:30–33; Appendicitis, 3:14; Cancer, 3:29–32; Gallstones, 3:58–59; Ulcer, peptic, 3:114–15
Storage of hazardous waste, 8:48
Storms, dangers of, 8:100–101
Strains. *See* Sprains and strains
Strangulated hernia, 3:76
Street violence, 8:92
Strength, 4:48–49, *99*, 100, 107
　weight training and, 4:132–33
　See also Exercise, 4:39–40; Fitness, 4:48–49
Strength exercise, 4:49, 100, 107, 108–9, *109*. *See also* Body building, 4:12–13
Strep throat, 2:86–87
Streptococcal infections, 2:86–87
　rheumatic fever following, 2:77–78
　See also Antibiotic treatment, 2:8–10; Bacterial infections, 2:13–15; Ear infections, 2:32–34; Impetigo, 2:49–50; Pneumonia, 2:72–73; Scarlet fever, 2:81–82; Sinusitis, 2:84–85; Sore throat, 2:85–86; Tonsillitis, 2:91–92
Streptococci, 2:13, 14
Stress, 1:7, 15–16, 38–39, 5:95–98
　anger and, 5:7, 8
　autonomic nervous system and, 5:15–16, *16*
　coping with, 5:29–30, 97–98
　disease and, 5:49, 97
　effects of, 3:38, 39, 89, 110, 114
　emotions and, 5:44
　fight-or-flight response to, 5:10, 16, 42
　friendships and, 5:47
　minor depression due to, 5:33
　noise pollution and, 8:59
　physiology of, 5:96

post-traumatic stress disorder, 5:12, 71–72
　prosocial behavior and, 5:74
　psychogenic amnesia and severe, 5:7
　psychosomatic disorders and, 5:78–79
　relaxation to reduce, 4:93, 94
　suicide and, 5:99, 100
　type A personality and, 5:70
　types of stressors, 5:95–96
Stress-management techniques, 5:29, 30, 97, 98–99
　relaxation training and, 5:30, 84, 97, 98–99
　See also Aerobic exercise, 4:4–6; Coping skills, 5:29–30
Stress response, 1:36
Stress test, 3:52, 106. *See also* Heart attack, 3:68–69; Heart disease, 3:69–72; Fitness training, 4:49–50
Stretching exercise, 4:40, 100, 109–10
　for flexibility, 4:50, 51–52
　See also Aerobic dance, 4:4; Fitness, 4:48–49; Running, 4:95–96
Striated muscles, 1:67
Stripping (removal of varicose veins), 3:116
Stroke, 1:21, 27, 49, 3:15, 19, 24, 106–8, *107*. *See also* Aneurysm, 3:13–14; Atherosclerosis, 3:19–20; Blood clot, 3:24; Diabetes, 3:46–48; Heart attack, 3:68–69; Hypertension, 3:77–78; Kidney disorders, 3:82–83; Paralysis, 3:95; Physical therapist, 9:30–31; Speech therapy, 9:40–41
Students Against Driving Drunk (SADD), 7:47
Stuttering, 3:104
Subaxillary temperature, 8:19
Subcutaneous injections, 7:67
Subcutaneous layer, 1:89–90
Subjective component of emotion, 5:42
Sublimation, 5:32
Sublingual glands, 1:86
Sublingual temperature, 8:19
Submandibular glands, 1:86
Substance Abuse and Mental Health Services Administration, 9:10. *See also* Preventive medicine, 9:34–35
Sucrose, 4:111
Sudden cardiac death, 3:71
Sudden infant death syndrome (SIDS), 3:108. *See also* Prenatal care, 6:78

Sugar, 4:110–11
artificial sweeteners substituting for, 4:8–9
as preservative, 4:52
as simple carbohydrate, 4:21
in soft drinks, 4:11
See also Carbohydrates, 4:21–22; Energy, food, 4:35–36; Fats, oils, and sweets group, 4:46–47; Fiber, 4:47–48; Overweight, 4:87; Starch, 4:106–7
Suicide, 5:99–100
depression and, 5:33, 99, 100
warning signs, 5:100
Suicide hot line, national, 5:100
Sulfa drugs, 7:96–97
Sulphur, 4:81
Sulphuraphane, 4:89
Sulphur dioxide, 8:7, 7
Sulphur oxides, 8:9–10, 91
Sun block, 7:97
Sunburn, 8:88
blisters, 3:23
Sun damage, 8:88–89
skin cancer and, 3:102, 103
sunscreens to prevent, 7:97, 8:89
See also Heatstroke, 8:49–50; Ozone, 8:64–65
Sun poisoning, 8:88
Sun Protection Factor (SPF), 7:97, 8:89
Sunscreens, 1:90, 7:97, 8:89. *See also* Skin cancer, 3:102–3
Sunstroke. *See* Heatstroke
Superego, 5:43
Superfund, 8:49, 89–90. *See also* Toxic substances, 8:91–92
Supination, 4:10
Support groups, 5:29–30
Suppository, 7:56
Suprarenal glands. *See* Adrenal glands
Supreme Court, medical ethics issues before, 9:21
Surgeon, 9:41
oral, 9:7
See also Surgery, 3:108–9; Physicians (M.D.'s), 9:31–34
Surgeon general on smoking, 7:98–99, 8:60
Surgery, 3:108–9
anesthesia during, 3:12–13, 109
anesthesiologist and, 9:4–5
for cancer, 3:30–31
coronary artery bypass, 3:19–20, 69, 73
heart, 3:73–74
laser, 3:83
plastic, 3:97
transplant, 3:113

weight loss through, 4:27–28
See also Surgeon, 9:41
Surgical amputation, 3:10–11
Surgical method of preventing pregnancy, 6:25
sterilization, 6:96–97
Surgical technologists, 9:23
Surrogate mother, 6:51, 9:22
Sutures, 1:91, *91*
Swallowing, 1:95
Sweat, 4:87–88, 101
antiperspirant to reduce, 7:42
dehydration and, 4:26, 88, 102
Sweat glands, 1:39, 89
boil as infection of, 2:15–16
Sweets. *See* Fats, oils, and sweets group
Swimmer's ear, 2:32, *33*
Swimming, 4:24, 112–13. *See also* Ear infections, 2:32–34; Hypothermia, 8:54–55
Swimming safety, 8:27, 98–99
Swollen glands, 1:64
Sybil, 5:65
Sydenham's chorea, 2:77
Sympathetic nerves, 1:73
Sympathetic nervous system, 1:7
emotion and, 5:42
stress and, 5:15–16, *16*
Symptothermal method of family planning, 6:66
Synapse, 1:72, 74
Synaptic knob, 1:74
Syncope. *See* Fainting
Synergism, drug, 7:48
Synovial membrane, 1:35, 58
Synovial sheaths, 1:28
Synovium, 1:56, 88, 3:16
Syphilis, 2:87–88, 6:*94*
organic brain disorders and, 5:66
reported cases of (1982–1990), 2:82
See also Lymphatic system, 1:63–64; Bacterial infections, 2:13–15; Chlamydial infections, 2:20–21; Gonorrhea, 2:41–42; Sexually transmitted diseases (STDs), 2:82, 6:94–95
Syrup of ipecac, 8:69
Systemic arteries, 1:12
Systemic circulation, 1:26
Systemic lupus erythematosus (SLE), 3:87
Systole, 1:48, *49*
Systolic pressure, 1:14–15, 3:77

Tachycardia, 8:72
Talus, 1:10

Tamoxifen, 7:22
Tampons, 6:34–35, 60
toxic shock syndrome and, 2:92, 93
Tanning salons, 8:88
Tapeworm, 2:88–89, *89*
Target heart rate, 4:6, 68
Target tissues (target organs), 1:35, 51
Tarsals, 1:41
Tars in tobacco, 7:98
Tartar (calculus), 1:29, 3:62, 7:100
Tartrazine, 4:53
Taste buds, 1:65, 86
Taxol, 7:23
Tay-Sachs disease, 3:110, 6:11, 42. *See also* Birth defects, 6:11–12; Genetic screening, 6:42–44; Genetic counselor, 9:12
TB. *See* Tuberculosis
TCAs (tricyclic antidepressants), 7:23
T cells, 1:13, 14, 54
HIV infection of, 2:5, 45–46, *46*
TCE (trichloroethylene), 8:*48*
Tea, 4:12
Team sports, 4:100
Tears, artificial, 7:58
Technologists and technicians, 9:15, 22–23
Teenage pregnancy, 6:97–98. *See also* Parenthood, 6:69–71; Child abuse, 8:22–23
Teeth. *See* Tooth
Television, violence on, 8:93
Temperature, body. *See* Body temperature
Temperature inversion, 8:90–91, *90*
air pollution and, 8:9, 90
Temperature method of family planning, 6:66
Temporal lobe, 1:21
Temporomandibular joint, 1:55, 3:*110*
Temporomandibular joint syndrome (TMJ), 1:55, 3:110–11. *See also* Jaw, 1:55; Arthritis, 3:15–17; Biofeedback, 5:18; Relaxation training, 5:84; Dental care, 9:7–8
Tendinitis, 1:28, 59, 3:111–12
sports and, 4:*103*, 104
See also Connective tissue, 1:27–28
Tendons, 1:28, 56
of elbow, 1:34–35
of hand, 1:46
of hip joint, 1:50
of knee, 1:58
in musculoskeletal system, 1:68, 69

Tendon transplants, 3:95
Tennis elbow, 1:35
Tension headache, 3:66
Terminally ill patients
    hospice for, 9:18–19
    right-to-die laws, 9:21
Testes (testicles), 1:36, *51, 82, 83,*
    6:79
    production of sperm in, 6:52–53
Testicular cancer, 6:18
Testicular self-examination, 6:18,
    98–99, *99. See also* Cancers of the
    sex organs, 6:17–18
Testing, medical, 9:22
Testosterone, 1:*51,* 6:52, 84–85
    anabolic steroids as synthetic
        variants of, 7:94–95
    hormone therapy with, 7:*64*
    puberty and, 6:79–80
Tetanus, 2:89–90
    DPT vaccine for, 2:31, 90, 100
Tetracyclines, 7:21
Tetrahydrocannabinol (THC), 7:71
Thalamus, 1:19, 5:42
Thalassemia, 3:12
Therapists, 9:15
    occupational, 9:26–27
    physical, 9:30–31
    psychotherapists, 9:35–36
Therapy. *See* Drug therapy, 5:39–40;
    Electroconvulsive therapy (ECT),
    5:41; Psychotherapy, 5:79–82; Hor-
    mone therapy, 7:63–64; Speech
    therapy, 9:40–41
Thermal inversion. *See* Temperature
    inversion
Thermal pollution, 8:91, 95. *See also*
    Sewage, 8:81–82; Water pollution,
    8:95–97
Thermal shock, 8:91
Thermometer, 8:57
    reading, 8:19, *19*
Thiamine, 4:116–17, *116, 121*
Thiopental, 7:32
Third-degree burns, 8:20, *20*
Thirst, 4:26–27, 88, 124
Thorax. *See* Chest
Three Faces of Eve, The, 5:65
Three Mile Island nuclear accident,
    8:62
Threshold dose, 7:45
Throat, 1:95–96, *95*
    laryngitis, 2:54–55
    sore, 2:85–86
    strep, 2:86–87
    See also Adenoids, 1:4–5; Diges-
        tive system, 1:30–33; Respira-
        tory system, 1:84–86; Tonsil,
        1:98

Throat culture, 2:28–29, 78, 86
Thrombophlebitis, 3:24, 34
Thrombosis, 3:24
Thrush, oral or genital, 2:19
Thunderstorms, 8:100
Thymus gland, 1:54
Thyroid disorders, 1:36–37, 3:112
Thyroid function tests, 3:112
Thyroid gland, 1:36, *51,* 70, 96–97, *97*
    overactive, 4:8
    See also Metabolism, 1:64–65;
        Thyroid disorders, 3:112
Thyroid hormone, 1:*51,* 96–97
Thyroid-stimulating hormone (TSH),
    1:36, *51,* 80
Thyroxine, 1:97, 4:27
Tibia, 1:10, 58
Ticks, 2:91, 8:17
    Lyme disease and, 2:58–59
    removal and treatment, 2:59, 91,
        91
    Rocky Mountain spotted fever
        and, 2:78
Tidal waves, 8:28
Timed specimen, 1:100
Time management, 5:29
Time-response relationship, 7:81
Tinnitus, 3:67
Tissue, 1:98
    scar, 1:86–87
    target, 1:35, 51
Tissue transplants, 3:113
Tobacco, 7:97–99
    chewing tobacco and snuff, 7:36
    the law and, 7:98–99, 8:60–61
    nicotine in, 7:9, 36, 85, 86, 92,
        96, 97, 98, 101
    other toxic substances in, 7:98
    quitting smoking, 7:85–87
    regulation of, 7:53
    smoking, 7:90–92
    See also Lung cancer, 3:85; Ad-
        diction, 7:4–5
Toddler stage, 1:24–25
Toenail, 1:69
    ingrown, 1:69, 3:57
Toes, 1:23, 41, 42
    Raynaud's phenomenon and,
        3:100
Tolerance, 5:40, 7:43, 99
    to alcohol, 7:12
    to barbiturates, 7:32
    to caffeine, 7:35
    to cocaine, 7:38
    to narcotics, 7:77
    psychoactive drug use and, 7:85
    stages of addiction, 7:4
    See also Alcoholism, 7:12–14;
        Drug use and abuse, 7:55–57

Tongue, 1:65
Tonometry test, 3:60
Tonsil, 1:98
    normal and infected, 2:*92*
    purpose of, 2:91
    See also Immune system,
        1:52–55; Tonsillitis, 2:91–92
Tonsillectomy, 1:98, 2:92
Tonsillitis, 1:98, 2:91–92. *See also*
    Abscess, 2:4; Rheumatic fever,
    2:77–78; Sore throat, 2:85–86
Tooth, 1:65, 99–100, *99*
    artificial teeth (dentures),
        3:45–46
    dental care for, 9:7–8
    dental problems and, 3:44–45, *44*
    gum disease and, 3:62–63
    orthodontic devices for teeth,
        3:45, 92, 111
    See also Dental examination,
        1:29; Jaw, 1:55; Mouth,
        1:65–66
Tooth decay, 3:44, 45
Toothpaste, 7:99–100. *See also* Dental
    problems, 3:44–45; Dental care,
    9:7–8
Tornadoes, 8:100
Touching, body language and, 5:19
Toxemia of pregnancy, 6:75
Toxic shock syndrome (TSS), 2:14,
    92–93, 6:18, 27, 29
    causes and treatment of, 2:93
    prevention of, 2:93
    use of tampons and, 6:35, 60
Toxic substances, 8:91–92
    carbon monoxide poisoning,
        8:21–22
    hazardous waste, 8:47–49
    lead, 8:56
    occupational injuries and ill-
        nesses from, 8:79
    oil spills, 8:63–64
    particulates, 8:65–66
    pollution from, 8:91, 95
    See also Acid rain, 8:6–7; Agri-
        cultural pollution, 8:7–8;
        Ozone, 8:64–65
Toxic waste dumps, Superfund and,
    8:89–90
Toxin, 2:94
    bacterial, 2:14
    See also Immune system,
        1:52–55; Antibody(ies), 2:10;
        Antigen, 2:10–11; Antiserum,
        2:11–12; Bacterial infections,
        2:13–15; Diphtheria, 2:30–31;
        Immunization, 2:47–49; Scar-
        let fever, 2:81–82; Tetanus,
        2:89–90

Toxoids, 2:48, 94
Toxoplasmosis during pregnancy, 6:12
Trace minerals, 4:79
Trachea (windpipe), 1:62, 70, 84, 95
Trachoma, 2:21
Traffic laws, 8:12, 14
Training
    assertiveness, 5:13
    cross, 4:24–25
    fitness, 4:49–50
    relaxation, 5:84
    social skills, 5:95
    for sports, 4:100–101
    strength, 4:107
    weight, 4:7, 12, 132–33
Trait theories, 5:69
Tranquilizers, 5:39, *39*, 7:87, 90
Transdermal patch, 7:83
Transfer, 5:57
Transfusion, blood, 3:25, 75
    Rh factor and reaction to, 6:82
Transient ischemic attacks (TIAs), 3:107
Transplant surgery, 3:113, 9:22
    bone marrow transplantation, 1:18–19, 3:84, 113
    dopamine-producing cells, 3:96
    heart, 3:72, 73–74
    immunosuppressant drug use after, 7:65
    kidney, 3:83
    nerve, 3:95
    non-Hodgkin's lymphoma and, 3:87
    tendon, 3:95
    See also Immune system, 1:52–55
Transsexuality, 6:99. *See also* Transvestism, 6:100
Transverse fracture, 8:42
Transvestism, 6:100. *See also* Gender identity, 6:38–40; Transsexuality, 6:99
Trapezius muscles, 1:88
Trauma center, 8:32
Traveler's diarrhea, 2:30, 4:58
Treadmills, 4:41–42
Tremors
    of earthquake, 8:28, 29
    Parkinson's disease and, 3:96
Trench mouth, 3:63
Treponema pallidum, 2:88
Tretinoin (Retin-A), 7:19
Tribadism, 6:47
Triceps muscles, 1:34, 35, 67, *67*
Trichinella spiralis, 2:94
Trichinosis, 2:94. *See also* Food poisoning, 4:57–58
Trichloroethylene (TCE), 8:48

Trichomonas vaginalis, 6:102
Trichomoniasis, 6:101, 102
Trichomoniasis protozoan, non-specific urethritis caused by, 2:67
Tricyclic antidepressants (TCAs), 7:23
Trifluridine, 7:29
Trigger points, 3:56
Trigger-point syndrome. *See* Fibrositis
Triiodothyronine, 1:97
Trimesters of pregnancy, 6:37–38, 74–75, *74*
Triplets, 6:62
Trip or tripping, 7:61, 71
Tris, 8:*48*
Trophic hormones, 1:35–36
Trust versus mistrust, 5:35
TSS. *See* Toxic shock syndrome (TSS)
TT (Text Telephone) telecommunications systems, 8:4
Tubal ligation, 6:25, 96, *96*
Tuberculin test, 2:95
Tuberculosis, 2:94–95, *95*
Tuber family, 4:107
Tumor, 3:25, 29, 114
    brain, 3:25–26
    See also Lymphatic system, 1:63–64; Breast cancer, 3:26–28; Cancer, 3:29–32
Twelve Steps of Alcoholics Anonymous, 7:9–10, *10*
Twins, 6:62
Tympanic membrane (eardrum), 1:34, 3:67
Type A personality, 5:7, 70, 97
Type B personality, 5:70, 97
Typhoid fever, 2:25, 96. *See also* Bacterial infections, 2:13–15; Immunization, 2:47–49; Salmonella infections, 2:80; Peritonitis, 3:97
Typhus, 2:96

Ulcer(s), 1:32, 65
    of herpes infections, 2:44
    peptic, 3:114–15, *115*
    See also Anemia, 3:11–12; Peritonitis, 3:97
Ulcerative colitis, 3:39
Ulna, 1:34, 35, *35*
Ultrasound, 6:100
    amniocentesis and, 6:43, 100
    prenatal care using, 6:78, 100
    See also X-ray examination, 3:117–18; Female reproductive system, 6:33–34

Ultraviolet (UV) radiation, 8:73, 74
    ozone layer and protection from, 8:10, 64, 65, 73
    sun damage from, 8:88–89
    sunscreens for protection against, 7:97, 8:89
Umbilical arteries, 6:101
Umbilical cord, 6:71, 101, *101*
    childbirth and, 6:21
    development of, 6:30
    percutaneous umbilical cord sampling, 6:44
    See also Amniotic fluid, 6:7; Female reproductive system, 6:33–34; Fetus, 6:37–38; Placenta, 6:71–72
Umbilical hernia, 3:76
Umbilical vein, 6:101
Unconscious mind, 5:31, 63
Undertows, swimming and danger of, 8:98
Underwater diving safety, 8:99
Underweight, 4:113, 128
    weight-gain strategy for, 4:128
    See also Weight assessment, 4:124–27
Unipolar depression. *See* Major depression
Universal choking sign, 8:24
Universal medical emergency identification symbol, 8:33
Unsaturated fats, 4:45–46
Ureter, 1:57, 101
    kidney stones in, 3:82
Urethra, 1:101, 6:53, 54
Urethritis. *See* Nonspecific urethritis
Urgicenters, 9:6
Uric acid crystals, buildup of, 3:17, 58
Urinalysis, 1:100. *See also* Liver, 1:60–62; Urinary tract, 1:100–101
Urinary incontinence, 3:80
Urinary tract, 1:100–101, *101. See also* Kidney, 1:57–58; Kidney disorders, 3:82–83
Urinary tract infection
    chlamydial, 2:20
    cystitis, 2:29
Urine, 1:57, 101
Urine test, 7:55
Urologists, 9:34
Urticaria (hives), 1:90, 3:6
Urushiol, 8:70
U.S. Department of Agriculture (USDA), 4:10, 29, 60
    Research Center on Aging, 4:89
U.S. Department of Health and Human Services, 4:29
Uterine cancer, 6:17

Uterus, **1**:83, 84, **6**:33
  hysterectomy and surgical removal of, **6**:48–49, *48*
  prolapsed, **6**:48

Vaccines
  antirabies, **2**:75
  BCG, **2**:95
  cholera, **2**:23
  as defense against bacterial infections, **2**:14–15
  DPT (diphtheria, pertussis, tetanus), **2**:31, 90, 100
  immunity and, **2**:47
  immunization with, **2**:47–49
  killed-virus, **2**:48
  live-virus, **2**:48
  MMR (measles, mumps, rubella), **2**:61, 66, 79
  against plague, **2**:71–72
  for pneumonia, **2**:73
  Sabin oral, **2**:74
  Salk, **2**:74
  smallpox, **2**:85
Vagina, **1**:83, **6**:33
Vaginal itching, **2**:54
Vaginal pouch, **6**:24
Vaginal thrush (vaginal yeast infection), **2**:19
Vaginismus, **6**:89
Vaginitis, **6**:101–2. *See also* Antibiotic treatment, **2**:8–10; Bacterial infections, **2**:13–15; Parasitic infections, **2**:68–69; Female reproductive system, **6**:33–34; Feminine hygiene, **6**:34–35
Values, **5**:100–101
  adult identity and, **5**:5
  changing, **5**:101
  conformity to peer group and, **5**:68
  development of, **5**:101
  See also Attitudes, **5**:13–14; Family, **5**:44–45; Responsibility, **5**:84–85
Valves, **1**:26
  in digestive system, **1**:31–32
  heart, **1**:48, 49, **3**:70, 73
  in veins, **1**:26, 102
Varicella. *See* Chicken pox
Varicella zoster (herpes zoster) virus, **2**:19
Varicose vein, **1**:102, **3**:34, 115–16. *See also* Circulatory system, **1**:25–27; Vein, **1**:102
Vas deferens, **6**:53, 96

Vasectomy, **6**:25, 96–97, *96*
Vasodilator drugs, **3**:19, 78, **7**:27
Vector-borne transmission of infection, **2**:51
Vegans, **4**:30, 113
Vegetables. *See* Fruits and vegetables group
Vegetarian diet, **4**:30–31, 72, 73, 113–15. *See also* Diets, **4**:30–32; Vitamin B complex, **4**:116–17
Vein(s), **1**:*26, 102, 102*
  diseases of, **3**:34, 115–16
  hepatic portal, **1**:61
  jugular, **1**:70
  pulmonary, **1**:26, 84, 102
  umbilical, **6**:101
  varicose, **3**:115–16
Venereal diseases. *See* Sexually transmitted diseases (STDs)
Venereal warts. *See* Genital warts
Venom allergies, **3**:6
Venous bleeding, **8**:18
Ventricles, **1**:26, 48, *49*, **3**:70
Ventricular fibrillation, **3**:71
Verbal aggression, **5**:5
Verbal communication, **5**:22
Verrucae, **2**:99
Vertebra(e), **1**:70, 93, 94, *94*
Vestibule, **1**:*33*, 34
Vestibulocochlear nerve, **3**:67
Vibrio cholerae, **2**:22
Vincent's disease. *See* Trench mouth
Vinyl chloride, **8**:*48*
Violence, **8**:92–93
  causes of, **8**:92–93
  child abuse, **8**:23
  kinds of, **8**:92
  physical, **5**:5
  preventing, **8**:93
  spouse abuse, **8**:86, 92, 93
  on television, **8**:93
  See also Aggressiveness, **5**:5–6; Sexual abuse, **6**:87
Violent pornography, **6**:72–73
Viral infections, **2**:97–98, **3**:30, 100
  body's response to, **2**:97–98
  chicken pox, **2**:19–20
  cold sore, **2**:23, 44
  common cold, **2**:23–24
  croup, **2**:27–28
  encephalitis, **2**:34
  genital warts, **2**:40, 99, 100
  influenza, **2**:52–53
  measles, **2**:60–61
  mononucleosis, **2**:65
  rabies, **2**:75
  treatment and prevention of, **2**:98, **7**:29–30
  yellow fever, **2**:25, 101

  See also Antibody(ies), **2**:10; Interferon, **2**:53–54; Microorganisms, **2**:63–65
Viral meningitis, **2**:61, 62
Virus(es), **1**:54, **2**:63, 97, *97*
  AIDS, **2**:5
  chronic fatigue syndrome and, **3**:38
  Epstein-Barr, **3**:38
  herpes simplex types 1 and 2, **2**:44, 97
  influenza, **2**:97, *97*
  pneumonia caused by, **2**:73
  poliomyelitis, **2**:73–74
  slow, **2**:97
  varicella (herpes) zoster, **2**:19
  warts caused by, **2**:99–100
Vision, peripheral, **3**:55, 60
Vision problems, **1**:41, **3**:116–17, *116*
  cataracts and, **3**:35–36
  eye tests for, **3**:55
  glaucoma and, **3**:60
  See also Eye, **1**:39–41; Eye disorders, **3**:54–55
Visiting nurses, **9**:18
Visual impairments, access for people with, **8**:4
Vitamin A, **4**:10, 65, 115–16, *121*
  deficiency, **4**:115
Vitamin B₆, **4**:*116*, 117, *121*
Vitamin B₁₂, **4**:114, *116*, 117, *121*
Vitamin B₁₂ (pernicious) anemia, **3**:12
Vitamin B complex, **4**:116–17, *116*. *See also* Anemia, **3**:11–12
Vitamin B deficiency, delirium tremens and, **7**:42
Vitamin C, **2**:24, **4**:52, 65, 117–18, *121*. *See also* Vitamin E, **4**:119–20
Vitamin D, **4**:114, 118–19, *121*
  deficiency, **1**:18
Vitamin E, **4**:52, 119–20, *121*. *See also* Vitamin C, **4**:117–18
Vitamin K, **4**:120–21, *121*
Vitamins, **4**:83, 84, 121–22, *121*
  fat-soluble, **4**:118, 119, 120, *121*, 122
  in fruits and vegetables, **4**:65
  in milk, **4**:77
  RDAs for, **4**:*121*, 122
  water-soluble, **4**:118, *121*, 122
Vitrification, **8**:49, 62
Vocal cords, **1**:96
Voluntary muscles, **1**:67
Vomiting, **2**:98–99
  induced after poisoning, **8**:69
  morning sickness, **2**:98, **6**:74
  See also Digestive system, **1**:30–33; Meningitis, **2**:61–62; Toxic shock syndrome (TSS),

2:92–93; Stomachache/indigestion, 3:105–6; Pregnancy, 6:74–76
Voyeurism, 6:9
Vulva, 6:33

Waist-to-hip ratio, 4:127
Waking consciousness, 5:63
Walking, 4:122–23. *See also* Athletic footwear, 4:9–10; Endurance, 4:34–35
Warts, 1:90, 2:99–100
  genital, 2:40, 99, 100, 6:*94*
  See also Viral infections, 2:97–98
Waste management, 8:93–94
  hazardous waste, 8:47–49
  recycling, 8:74–76, 85–86
  sewage treatment, 8:82
  solid waste, 8:84–86
  See also Air pollution, 8:9–10; Sanitation, 8:80–81; Toxic substances, 8:91–92; Water pollution, 8:95–97
Wastewater. *See* Sewage
Water, 4:11, 123–24
  balance of, 4:124
  electrical safety and, 8:30
  fluid replacement during sports, 4:102
  foods with high water content, 4:123
  See also Beverages, 4:10–12; Body metabolism, 4:15–17; Dehydration, 4:26–27; Minerals, 4:79–81; Diuretic, 7:44–45
Water conservation, 8:94–95. *See also* Agricultural pollution, 8:7–8; Thermal pollution, 8:91; Water pollution, 8:95–97; Water purity, 8:97–98; Weather-related emergencies, 8:99–101
Water pollution, 8:95–97
  acid rain and, 8:6–7
  agricultural chemicals and, 8:8, 95, 96
  ecosystem upset by, 8:29
  oil spills and, 8:40, 63–64
  preventing or reducing, 8:94–95, 97
  sanitation and, 8:80
  sewage and, 8:81–82
  thermal pollution, 8:91
  types of, 8:95, *96*
  water purity and, 8:97–98
  See also Toxic substances, 8:91–92

Water purity, 8:97–98. *See also* Agricultural pollution, 8:7–8; Sewage, 8:81–82; Water conservation, 8:94–95; Water pollution, 8:95–97
Water safety, 8:98–99
  prevention of drowning, 8:27, 98–99
  See also Accidents, 8:5–6
Watersheds, 8:94
Water-soluble vitamins, 4:118, *121*, 122
Water treatment, 8:97
Watson, John B., 5:77
Weather conditions, auto safety and, 8:13
Weather-related emergencies, 8:99–101
  earthquakes, 8:27–29
  hypothermia, 8:54–55
Weight assessment, 4:124–27, *125*
  methods of, 4:125–27
  obesity and, 4:85–86
  for overweight, 4:87
  for underweight, 4:113
  See also Body composition, 4:13–14; Diets, 4:30–32; Eating disorders, 4:33–34; Fitness, 4:48–49; Weight-gain strategy, 4:128; Weight-loss strategy, 4:128–30
Weight-gain strategy, 4:30, 113, 128
  for underweight, 4:113
  See also Body metabolism, 4:15–17; Fats, oils, and sweets group, 4:46–47; Weight assessment, 4:124–27; Weight management, 4:130–32
Weight lifting, 4:108
Weight-loss quackery, 9:38
Weight-loss strategy, 4:128–30, *129*
  diet aids for, 4:27–28
  diet foods for, 4:29–30
  diets for, 4:30
  diet success rates, 4:*129*
  elements of successful, 4:129–30
  fad diets and, 4:42–43, 130
  for overweight, 4:87, 128–30
  strategies to avoid, 4:130
  to treat obesity, 4:86, 128
  See also Weight assessment, 4:124–27; Weight management, 4:130–32
Weight machines, 4:42
Weight management, 4:130–32
  body metabolism and, 4:16, 17
  diets and, 4:30–32
  eating right for, 4:131–32

energy-balance equation and, 4:21, 36, 131
excess body fat and, 4:13
exercise for, 4:132
food energy and, 4:35–36
See also Energy, physical, 4:36–38; Lifestyle, 4:71–72; Risk factors, 4:94–95
Weight training, 4:7, 12, 132–33. *See also* Endurance, 4:34–35; Fitness, 4:48–49; Strength, 4:107
Wellness, 4:133. *See also* Preventive medicine, 9:34–35
Western blot analysis, 2:6
Wet dream. *See* Nocturnal emission
Wet gangrene, 3:59
Wet pleurisy, 3:98
Wheelchairs, access for, 8:4–5
White blood cells (leukocytes), 1:12, 13, *13*, 18, 53, 100
  abnormal, 3:83
  antibodies produced by, 2:10
  infection-fighting, 2:37
  mononucleosis virus in, 2:65
  in pus, 2:74
Whiteheads, 3:4
White matter, 1:93
White rice, 4:17
Whole-grain breads, 4:17
Whooping cough, 2:100
  DPT vaccine for, 2:31, 90, 100
  See also Pneumonia, 2:72–73
Will, living, 9:21, 29
Williams-Steiger Occupational Health and Safety Act (1970), 8:63
Wilson's disease, 3:38
Windpipe (trachea), 1:62, 70, 84, 95
Wisdom teeth, impacted, 3:45
Withdrawal syndrome, 7:100–101
  addiction and, 7:4–5, 57
  from alcohol, 7:9
  from amphetamines, 7:15
  from barbiturates, 7:32
  from caffeine, 7:35, 101
  delirium tremens (DTs) and, 7:42
  during detoxification, 7:14, 50
  in fetal alcohol syndrome baby, 7:58
  from heroin, 7:62–63, 101
  from narcotics, 7:77, 101
  quitting smoking and, 7:86
  from sedatives, 7:88
  symptoms of, 7:101
  treatment of, 7:101
  See also Alcoholics Anonymous (AA), 7:9–12; Drug rehabilitation, 7:49–50; Hangover, 7:61–62

Women
cancers of sex organs in, 6:17
condoms for, 6:24
effect of steroid use on, 7:95
fertility testing of, 6:51
hormone therapy for, 7:63–64
infertility in, 6:50–51
sexual dysfunction in, 6:89
Women smokers, 7:91
Workplace, sex roles in, 6:86
Workplace safety. *See* Safety on the job
World Health Organization (WHO), 2:60, 85
Worldwatch Institute, 8:35
Worms, parasitic, 2:64
Wounds, 8:101
from animal bites, 8:16
first aid for, 8:18, 101
minor and severe, 8:55

See also Tetanus, 2:89–90; Bites and stings, 8:15–18; Injuries, 8:55–56
Wrist, carpal tunnel syndrome and, 3:34–35
Wrist joint, 1:46
Wundt, Wilhelm, 5:76

X chromosome, 6:40, 42
Xiphoid process, 1:24
X-ray examination, 3:40, 117–18
chest, 2:72, 95
dental X rays, 1:29
exposure to radiation through, 8:73
for fracture, 8:42
precautions with, 8:74
See also CAT scan, 3:36; Radiation therapy, 3:99; Mammogram, 6:54–55; Radiologist, 9:38–39

Y chromosome, 6:40, 42
Yeast breads, 4:17
Yeast infection, vaginal, 2:19
Yeasts, 2:64
Yellow fever, 2:25, 101
Yersinia pestis, 2:71
Yin and yang, 4:73, 73
Young adulthood, 5:5
Yo-yo syndrome, 4:42, 130

Zen macrobiotic diet, 4:73
Zidovudine (AZT), 2:7, 7:29, 30, 31
Zinc, 4:80, 81
Zygote, 6:35, 36, 40